Los Altos Methodist
Church Library

# SIXTY-PLUS&FIT AGAIN

# SIXTY-PLUS

# & FIT AGAIN

613.7
R6

## EXERCISES FOR OLDER MEN AND WOMEN

# Magda Rosenberg

### Physician's Foreword by I. Rossman, M.D.

*Illustrations by Hoke Wilson*

M. EVANS AND COMPANY, INC. / NEW YORK, N. Y. 10017

Los Altos Methodist
Church Library

3421

M. Evans and Company titles are distributed in
the United States by the J. B. Lippincott Company,
East Washington Square, Philadelphia, Pa. 19105;
and in Canada by McClelland & Stewart Ltd.,
25 Hollinger Road, Toronto M4B 3G2, Ontario

**Library of Congress Cataloging in Publication Data**
Rosenberg, Magda.
  Sixty-plus and fit again.

  1. Exercise.  2. Aged—Care and hygiene.
I. Title.
RA781.R68     613.7'1'0240565     76-49130
ISBN 0-87131-224-7
ISBN 0-87131-237-9 Paperback

Copyright © 1977 by Magda Rosenberg
All rights reserved under International and Pan-
American Copyright Conventions

Design by Joel Schick

Manufactured in the United States of America

9 8 7 6 5 4 3 2 1

To all the senior citizens I know and to my family: Marty, June, David, Mark, Maury and Rose.

## ACKNOWLEDGMENTS

I could not have written this book without the inspiration and help of thousands of senior citizens in my community and in my classes who have taught me as much as I have taught them. I also appreciate the help of Joyce S. Christmas in preparing this book.

# Contents

# *Foreword*

*U*NTIL recent years, the many benefits of exercise were not fully appreciated, even in medical circles—doctors themselves were often unflattering examples of the effects of sedentary living. We now know that exercise programs can be of inestimable value; they have reached the status of medical prescription for some disorders, for example, chronic backache, certain forms of heart disease, and chronic fatigue states. We are still far from knowing the full impact of year-in, year-out exercise on human beings, but many doctors have been impressed by the truth behind the generalization that no marathon runner has ever died of a heart attack.

In fact, it was nationwide concern over the dramatic increase in heart disease in recent decades that led to an examination of a sedentary life pattern as a contributing factor. Older citizens who can remember back to the early years of this century can testify that heart attacks were not the everyday occurrence they are today. Significantly (and difficult to believe from our present vantage point), the *first* description of a coronary thrombosis in American medical literature was written in 1912 by an observant Chicago physician.

We all know that labor-saving devices have dominated the twentieth century, and never more so than in the past few decades: the automobile, the washing machine, the vacuum cleaner, the power lawn mower, even the electric egg beater and can opener. The resulting decrease in the use of our muscles in the simple matters of everyday living means, of course, less exercise for the heart muscle. This is true for the young as well as the elderly.

Some individuals have realized with a start that their muscles have become weak and shrunken, that their wind is bad. They seek to remedy their deficiency with vigorous exercise, but it seems to me most unlikely that playing tennis once a week can substitute for day-in, day-out exercise; and I do not recommend the most vigorous of exercises, jogging, for my older patients unless they are long-time joggers. I do believe, however, that a daily pattern of mild to moderate exercise is desirable and beneficial for all age groups. When it comes to older persons, those for whom *Sixty-Plus and Fit Again* is intended, the question is: How beneficial?

Any doctor who has worked with older people can attest to the value of exercise, whether for a special purpose such as recovery of a lost function or for maintenance of general fitness and energy levels. "Atrophy of disuse" is a well-known term in geriatric medicine; it specifies a shrinkage of muscles and the weakness that follows as a consequence of non-use. Such atrophy also affects the joints the muscles act upon, so that stiffness of the joint and even severe limitation of motion (contracture) can result.

It is always an impressive demonstration of the body's power to heal and return to normal to follow the effect of regular exercise on both the weak muscle and the contracture. With sensible exercise (no rush, no pushing the body past the pain point), the muscle becomes bigger and stronger; the joint develops a full range of motion. Many older, sedentary people have allowed themselves to fall into the condition where muscles are weak from disuse and easily fatigued. Stiffness and decreased mobility of joints are too readily attributed to "age" or "arthritis," when in fact it is poor conditioning, which is often promptly reversed by exercise.

Our society, never kind to the old, has not paid much heed to the exercise needs of the senior-age groups. We see public playgrounds for children and tennis courts for younger adults, but little or no space and programming are devoted to older persons. Most senior citizens centers have also been neglectful, perhaps reflecting the false but widespread notion that physical activity is only for the young and strong.

It is to Mrs. Rosenberg's credit that she has chosen to work with senior citizens in this neglected area. She recognizes the need for exercise adapted to the requirements of life-cycle changes, and she has demonstrated with graphic examples the desirable impact and therapeutic value of exercise for those in the older age groups.

Exercising with a group has social value; it is more fun. But in the final analysis, exercise is a necessity, to be done without fail, even if, like brushing one's teeth, one does it alone. As Mrs. Rosenberg points out, only a few minutes a day are all that is needed to maintain fitness and prevent atrophy in senior citizens.

A few minutes a day seems like a small investment for a rich return. A regular exercise program gives a sense of well-being in the present, and it also gives the older person a reserve of strength to call upon if the need arises. From the viewpoint of the physician, this physical reserve in a patient, especially an older one, can be critical: it may determine whether one becomes bedbound or bounces back after a fracture, an operation, a bout of the flu. Many experiences in this area have convinced me of the value of exercise.

*Sixty-Plus and Fit Again* makes an important contribution to this end. Mrs. Rosenberg's experience in the implementation of fitness programs for older adults is apparent throughout this book. It requires patience and intelligent observation to develop a therapeutic philosophy such as Mrs. Rosenberg possesses. The care and thoughtfulness of her approach makes her book safe and useful for older people, and those who work with them, in increasing overall fitness and health.

*Isadore Rossman, M.D., Ph.D.*

# SIXTY-PLUS & FIT AGAIN

# ONE

# *Why Exercise?*

**W**HAT would it be worth to you to be independent as long as you live? To be able to take care of yourself without the help of anyone else, to come and go with freedom, to feel well and look well? What would it be worth to know that your later years can be as full of activity, interest, and enjoyment as your youth and middle age?

You have already spent a good many years of your life being responsible for others: raising children, caring for a home and family, working to support dependents, perhaps even caring for elderly parents. Over the years, your responsibilities have diminished: the children are grown and gone from home, you have reached retirement age, you may be alone in the world. Without realizing it you may, in turn, be getting more and more dependent on the help of others just to survive. You don't feel able to get out and around any more. Each day finds you a little less active. You are tired, your body is weaker, you are—old.

What is old age?

Old age is when your physical impairment dictates your life.

Old age is when the respect you have earned is denied you because you have become a burden and a threat to younger generations, when you are dependent and helpless.

But that kind of old age is not inevitable. If you are a senior citizen, it is up to you, now, to decide what your later years are going to mean to you.

You can sit in your armchair, looking at the four walls or your television set. You can allow disabilities to rule your life. You can withdraw from the world outside and let your body and mind go to sleep. Or you can do something about it.

All it takes is a few minutes a day to feel younger, look younger, regain the energy you had to do what you want to do now.

I'm not talking about a magic formula or a mysterious secret. There's no secret and no mystery to this fountain of youth. You can find it with a little will power and a little knowledge.

I'm talking about *exercise*. A few minutes of exercise a day can mean the difference between an unhappy and dependent old age, and later years that are full of pleasure and activity—and usefulness. Only minutes a day, every day, can turn a healthy senior citizen who has succumbed to a sedentary life into an active, vigorous human being who can prove to the world that old age does not mean the end of living.

## Looking Back

Look back for a minute on your younger years. Look at the younger people around you. For a good portion of all our lives, it seems, we are constantly fatigued, tense, filled with aches and pains. We get up in the morning feeling listless and stripped of energy, wishing we could turn back the clock and spend a few more minutes in bed. We fall asleep at our desks and are revived by periodic coffee breaks. We send the children out to play and wonder where we are going to get the strength to clean the house and do the laundry.

All our lives, we have not exercised properly. Young men and women in their twenties and thirties; executives and homemakers in their forties and fifties; office and factory workers, professional people, senior citizens of sixty, seventy, eighty, and older—all of us in every part of society, through ignorance or perhaps laziness, allow ourselves to be ruled, and overcome, by our bodies.

As we grow older, the muscles of our body grow weaker from lack of use. And the symptoms of not using our muscles properly reveal themselves in fearful proportions the older we get. The sedentary senior citizen who has neglected his or her body through all those years of youth and middle age becomes, at worst, a vegetable, the victim of his or her own negligence. In the process, the senior citizen loses the respect and sympathy of younger society, which sees its own future in the aged and does not like what it sees.

Our youth- and beauty-oriented society still does not understand properly the role of exercise in keeping us fit and active through all the years of our lives. Yet muscle tone, flexibility of joints, and the circulatory functions responsible for the stimulation of mind and body cannot be achieved without motion: controlled exercise in a program designed to keep every part of the body in good working order. Teenagers may tell you that they take part in sports because it makes their parents proud of them or because they want to get athletic scholarships to college. Never, it seems, is the relationship between physical activity and health made clear. That lack of education, starting at a very young age, is the reason why we turn human beings into human waste in older citizens.

"But," you may ask, "why should *I* exercise? I'm getting on in years—I may not have many years left. Why should I bother?"

My answer to that is, "Who are you to say how many years lie ahead? Who am I to put a number to them?"

I remember reading a newspaper report of a party held to celebrate the one hundredth birthday of a woman who was interviewed for the occasion.

When asked about the joys and regrets of her life, she said, "When I was eighty, my son offered to buy me new dentures, but I told him not to bother. At eighty I probably didn't have much longer, and it would just be a waste of money. Now here I am twenty years later, still without those dentures. If I had it all to do over again, I'd have said yes to my son. How did I know how long I would last?"

That is why you should exercise, whatever your age may be. It is never too late to take advantage of what life has to offer. It is not too late now for you to learn to be in control of your body, to make it work for you and not against you in the years to come. In the following chapters, you will find the exercise program you need, the do's and don'ts, and the reasons why exercise can be the most important minutes-a-day investment you can make.

I have seen over and over again how exercise gives senior citizens healthy bodies and new beauty. I have seen thousands of minds stimulated and a new interest in living reborn in people in their seventies, eighties, and even nineties. Exercise did it for them, and it can do the same for you.

## *Your Responsibility*

As a senior citizen, you have a continuing responsibility to younger generations that does not decrease along with your day-to-day obligations to others.

You must prove to younger people that old age is not a time to be feared. It is a time of pride, dignity, and well-earned enjoyment of life. You can educate others by your example; you can prove to your sons and daughters and grandchildren that the later years can be as stimulating and interesting as the years of youth.

It is alarming, as we get older, how a simple act like sitting down in a chair or getting into a car becomes a physical struggle. Older people know this; younger people can see it happening. But it doesn't need to be so. Fingers that can barely pick up a spoon because the muscles have wasted away from lack of use can be made useful again with the proper exercise. A fatiguing walk of half a block can become the first leg of a ten-block stroll to visit family and friends. Backs don't have to ache, legs don't have to be weak. Life doesn't have to be a tedious, lonely existence because of physical impairment. You don't have to sit in a chair alone at home, an object of pity to your offspring, someone's unwanted responsibility.

Too many senior citizens accept physical and mental crippling as an inevitable part of old age. Too many younger people accept that state in their elders as inevitable. In desperation, too many aged give up on life and find solace in a rocking chair, and their children and grandchildren allow them to do so.

How can we put a stop to that despair, that waste of important and useful human beings?

If there is nothing medically wrong with you, but you find that your body is going downhill through a lack of exercise, the answer is a physical fitness program: regular, controlled exercise, suited to the special needs of the senior citizen.

A program of physical fitness—at any age, but especially for the senior citizen—can mean the difference between a healthy, active life and a living death. I am going to show you how to do it. I'm going to show you what exercise has done for others like you, and I'm going to tell you how to make it work for you. All you need is the determination to make the most of what this book has to offer.

When you have finished reading and have begun your exercise program, you will have the answer to the question, "Why exercise?"

For independence, for health, for beauty. To prove that usefulness does not end with retirement, when the house is empty of children, when a person becomes a "senior citizen."

Whatever your age, there are years of living ahead of you. What you do with them depends on you.

# TWO

# *Encouragements and Warnings*

---

"T ODAY I said goodbye to a very old friend of mine: my cane," Mr. Kraft told me one day at the end of an exercise class. Mr. Kraft is ninety-four.

Minnie, a widow in her seventies, rarely left her house when I first met her, "because," she explained, "every time I had to go around the corner, I got exhausted, so I ended up taking taxis when I had to go anywhere. That got too expensive, and I lost confidence in my ability to get around on foot alone. Finally I just stayed home."

Until she joined a senior citizens exercise class and built up the strength and energy to walk for miles.

"Not only do I feel a hundred percent more agile these days," she says, "but I've even lost inches. I'm a whole size smaller!"

"Before I started doing your exercises to strengthen my fingers," seventy-five-year-old Anna told me, "I couldn't hold a cup of coffee in my hands. Every time I picked up the cup, my hand was so weak I always spilled it."

Anna was sitting at a table with two friends and me at the

senior citizens hotel where she lives. We were all having coffee, and Anna's hand was as steady as mine.

"It was an embarrassment for me to sit like this with friends," Anna said. "I kept dropping the cup. These ladies remember—" Anna's friends both nodded.

"It embarrassed us, too," one said. "Sometimes we'd look for ways to get out of sitting down with Anna."

"Well," said Anna, "since you educated me to the fact that my hands could be made stronger with exercise, look at me! I haven't dropped a cup in weeks. I enjoy being with my friends again. It may not seem like much to a kid like you," she said to me seriously, "but for me it's almost a miracle."

Anna, Mr. Kraft, Minnie, and thousands of others have joined in my exercise classes for senior citizens. They came walking slowly and with difficulty, with their muscles weak from lack of use—years of it. They came with canes, with hands that couldn't hold a cup, with legs that wouldn't carry them half a block to the grocery store. Many of them were unconvinced that a safe and sound exercise program would benefit them at all.

"We're old," they said. "Our doctors have told us we're not sick, just old. There's nothing to be done. Our children tell us we're old, we should take it easy."

"Old age to my son," one man told me, "means that I shouldn't move a muscle. I should just sit there in my armchair and watch myself die. But I don't feel like dying yet. What can I do?"

I tell them there is something they *can* do. Their doctors are wrong, their children and grandchildren are wrong, society is wrong. And you are going to prove them wrong. In this book, you are going to learn how to exercise.

## Your Body

The human body is made of bones and blood vessels and organs and muscles—muscle, in fact, makes up more than half of the body. Imagine what happens if more than half the body is rarely used, rarely put into motion through exercise. Imagine what happens to your body if you sit in a chair day after day and never move a muscle.

You have all seen what happens to an arm that has been broken and put into a cast for weeks. It doesn't matter if that arm belongs to a sixty-year-old grandmother or a ten-year-old boy. When it comes out of the cast, the muscles that haven't been used for weeks are weak. They have to be exercised back to health. After a broken hip or leg has mended and the cast is off, you have to have exercise therapy to bring the muscles in the limb back to normal.

The muscles of an older person which have not been used for years are like the muscles in that broken arm or leg. They have grown weak from lack of use; they must be brought back to a normal state through exercise.

It will not be easy, after so many sedentary years, to bring your whole body back. Weak muscles, stiff joints, the physical impairment that comes not from illness but from neglect, aren't overcome overnight. It takes will power and determination to change your lifestyle to one that includes regular exercise. You will be tempted to make excuses to yourself when you don't feel like exercising: "I'm too tired today." "Nothing will help me any more." "I'm too old to bother."

Age has nothing to do with it. Our muscles don't know the difference between old and young. In one of my classes for younger people, Marie was my star performer. She was a lovely, athletic young woman in her late twenties, and she often said that going without exercise even for a single day made her feel tense and out of sorts. Her trim, healthy body was a perfect advertisement for the benefits of regular exercise.

One day I brought a large ball to the class and started throwing it back and forth to the students as a warmup exercise. The first time I threw the ball to Marie, she dropped it. I tried again, and again she dropped it. I was puzzled. Why couldn't that physically fit young woman seem to grasp the ball?

Then I noticed something about Marie that I hadn't seen before. She had the most beautiful long fingernails I had ever seen. That alone shouldn't have prevented her from catching a ball, but something else did: she lived in fear of chipping or breaking her nails. As a result, she confessed that she rarely used her fingers. The muscles of her body were strong and healthy and magnificently toned—except for the muscles of her fingers. They had deteriorated from lack of use to the point where that woman in her twenties was unable to control them.

"Marie," I told her, "you are going to have to make the choice between saving your nails and saving your fingers. You know enough about exercise to know this is true."

Marie admitted that I was right, and chose to save her fingers, giving up her long nails and beginning a program of finger exercises.

If that was true for a young woman, how much worse is it for an older person who has allowed *all* the muscles of the body to deteriorate through long years of inactivity?

Perhaps, if you are forty or fifty years older than Marie, her story hasn't convinced you. After all, she wasn't a senior citizen like you. But what about Mrs. Koster, the victim of a broken leg late in her sixties? To me, she is the perfect example of what can be accomplished with exercise.

I met Mrs. Koster by chance one day while I was taking a walk through the town where I live. I particularly noticed her because, of all things, she was walking along a busy downtown street in the gutter instead of on the sidewalk. I could see that she was not young, and that she was walking with some difficulty. Because of my interest in the lives of senior citizens, I stopped and asked her why she was walking in the street and not on the sidewalk.

Mrs. Koster looked at me with some embarrassment and said, "I'm walking in the gutter because I just can't lift my feet up to get on the curb. It's terrible to get old and weak."

She refused my offer of help and walked on past me around the corner, still in the street. It was only a moment later that a young bicyclist rounded the corner behind her at full speed, and Mrs. Koster was on the ground with a broken leg.

The next time I saw Mrs. Koster was months later, at one of my senior citizens exercise classes.

"Do you see this leg?" she said. "It's the one that was broken that day in the street. It was in a cast for weeks, and when the cast finally came off, it was so weak I couldn't stand on it. So the doctors gave me exercises for it, and I did them faithfully every day. Well, it worked. Watch this."

Mrs. Koster proceeded to lift the leg up—and up, and up. She lifted it up to her ear!

"That's what exercise can do," she said. "That leg is about forty years younger than the rest of my body. Look."

She could barely raise her other leg, the one that was not impaired and had not been exercised, off the floor.

"This other leg is as old as I am. The one that was broken is like a kid next to his grandfather. So I'm here to do for the rest of my body what exercise did for that leg."

Mrs. Koster's example set the class working hard at their exercises. Mrs. Koster herself, knowing from personal experience what exercise can do, was the most avid participant of all.

Senior citizens have to defend themselves constantly against society, the self-appointed guardians of the aged who see old age as total disability. A while ago, someone discovered that there was an 104-year-old man living by himself. He cooked for himself, he shopped for himself, he took care of himself completely, without help. Society was shocked. A man of 104 couldn't possibly be able to care for himself. He should immediately be put into a senior citizens home to be taken care of by others. Then they brought television cameras into his little room, and he demonstrated how he was able to be self-sufficient and agile at his age. The answer was exercise. He had been faithfully doing daily exercises that kept his muscles in tone, his body flexible, his blood circulating, and his mind alert.

Society has come to look upon older people as useless entities. It wants to help them, when they can help themselves; it wants to tell them that there is no hope. How often do I hear from older people, "We're old, our doctors tell us we're old. Society tells us we're old and have no reason for living. There's nothing that will help us."

Alas, most doctors do not have the special education required to understand geriatric needs—specifically, the kind of physical impairment that comes from allowing the body to deteriorate through lack of use and not from illness. Most of us look up to our doctors as the ultimate healers and savers of lives. If we display the disabilities that can accompany old age, and yet there is nothing organically wrong and no reason for hospitalization, the solution all too often may be a lot of pills to be taken at different hours of the day.

"I'm so mixed up with my little rainbow-colored box," Louise told me, "that I don't know whether I should take the pink pill at three o'clock, the red pill at four o'clock, or the little white pill at two o'clock. All I know is that ever since I started taking all these pills, I feel like I'm on a merry-go-round that makes me dizzy and that's all. All those pills certainly don't make me feel any better, and all the doctor says is, 'Take it easy.' "

The saddest prescription I know for older people is, "Take it easy."

My friend Mr. Malone, who's close to eighty, told me, "My doctor keeps on assuring me that there is nothing he can do for me any more. He tells me, 'Mr. Malone, you are an old man. What do you expect me to do—make you young again?' Of course I don't expect that, but if I can see what exercise does for me and my friends, why can't he?"

There is such ambivalence toward doctors among the older people I meet every day that I hear jokes about it all the time. Mr. Malone loves to tell one that isn't so far from the truth.

"I called my doctor last week and said, 'Doctor, everything in my body hurts. My head aches, I see spots in front of my eyes. I have to see you right away.' And the doctor said, 'But Mr. Malone, we're very busy. We can't give you an appointment until next week.'

"So I said to the doctor, 'You've told me I'm an old man. A week from now I may be dead.' And the doctor answered, 'Well, Mr. Malone, if you are dead, we'll cancel the appointment.'"

Mr. Malone's joke is always greeted with laughter by his fellow senior citizens. They've all had similar experiences. There are too few doctors, or for that matter too few people anywhere in society, who understand the aged—too few who understand that besides pills to cure disease, there are other ways to cure aches and pains caused by muscles weakened from lack of use.

The doctor is often the last resort of older people. He is the one who, it seems, can promise us life or death. Doctors should —indeed, I believe, *must*—be trained to understanding; they must learn that there is hope, genuine hope, for senior citizens.

They must be able to say with conviction, "There is something you can do. You can go home and walk, exercise, bring your body back to condition, build up your strength with activity." What hope, what a psychological boost lie in those few words, and what possibilities for senior citizens who take them to heart and undertake an exercise program!

## Exercise and Aging

It is important that you yourself understand the reasons for regular exercise. Only then will you be exercising with a purpose in mind. That purpose has nothing to do with beauty, although that is the usual argument for getting people exercising, and it has everything to do with health. There are a few pioneers in the medical profession who understand why you, as senior citizens, can't make a better investment in time and energy than exercise.

The President's Council on Physical Fitness wrote in *Adult Physical Fitness:*

> There is strong authoritative support for the concept that regular exercise can help prevent degenerative disease and *slow down the physical deterioration that accompanies aging.*
>
> The evidence is conclusive: individuals who consistently engage in proper physical activity have better job performance records, fewer degenerative diseases, and *probably a longer life expectancy than the population at large. By delaying the aging process, proper exercise also prolongs your active years.* [author's italics]

Remaining fit and active through exercise can aid in preventing aging; it can retard some of the aspects of old age which make the later years loom up as a terrifying stretch of time filled only with aches and pains, confinement to the home, loneliness, and unhappiness.

"Medical research," writes Dr. Kenneth Cooper in *Aerobics,* "has given us new insight into the process of aging. Aging is accelerated by inactivity. Lack of exercise seems to be a major factor in premature aging."

A leisurely, inactive existence, the silent crippler that so many of us look forward to in our old age, is fast becoming the disease of our times. People of all ages ignore the benefits of exercise—except for the promises of sudden beauty that catch the interest for a time. However, a former president of the American Medical Association has said, "It begins to appear that exercise is the master conditioner for the healthy and the major therapy for the ill." Other medical researchers tell us that "exercise is medically approved as one of our greatest weapons against illness and premature aging."

"Disuse," says "The Fitness Challenge in the Later Years,"

prepared by the President's Council on Physical Fitness and Sports and the Administration on Aging, "is the mortal enemy of the human body. We know today that how a person lives, not how long he lives, is responsible for many of the physical problems associated with advanced age."

Dr. Paul Dudley White, whose far-ranging interests in many areas of medicine included the benefits of exercise (including his own widely publicized bicycle-riding activities at an advanced age), warns us of the "swelling of the legs, fatigue of muscles, blood clotting and many other ills sedentary existence may bring." Dr. White reports that there is evidence that exercising the leg muscles may have a retarding or even preventive effect on the early development of hardening of the arteries, which is now one of the most common and serious diseases in this country.

With the evidence in favor of exercise that is piling up, it would appear that it would be simple to preserve the body throughout our lives just by keeping fit. That would eliminate many problems in later years; the exercise habit would be so strong at every age that maintaining physical fitness would be as ordinary as driving a car or going to work every morning.

Unfortunately, we have a way of turning our backs on preventive action and waiting instead until a problem occurs. Only then do we try to reverse it.

Mr. Foster spent his whole life cooped up in his little grocery store. Any day of the week I could find him there, devoting all his time to his business and otherwise not active. Over the years, I saw him gain weight and grow older-looking. All his friends and customers were saddened one day to hear that he had had a heart attack.

A while later I was surprised to see a thinner, healthier-looking Mr. Foster walking briskly in my direction.

We stopped to chat, and Mr. Foster said, "It's funny. Had I cared about myself a little more, that heart attack might not have happened. Now my doctor has impressed on me the need to get out and walk to keep my heart in good working order. But all those years I sat in the grocery store, no one could have convinced me that one day I would be exercising for my health —*after* it was almost too late for me.  It should have been the other way around—exercise *before* it was too late."

"All right," you may agree, "Mr. Foster was convinced, but I'm not. What can it really do for me or my friends who may already have some disabilities? What about arthritis, for example?"

Many of my arthritic students tell me how much better they feel after gentle, well-supervised motions. Of course, if you are afflicted with arthritis, you should do no exercises unless they have been approved by your doctor. But see what appears in a booklet entitled "Arthritis, the Basic Facts," published by The Arthritis Foundation:

> Much of the crippling by rheumatoid arthritis develops because painful joints have been kept for long periods in what feels like a comfortable position. They then have stiffened, become "frozen," and muscles around the joints have become weak from inactivity. The way to keep joints mobile is to move them.
>
> "Exercise" for rheumatoid arthritis does not mean athletics, or lifting heavy things, or doing anything strenuous. Each patient is given special "quiet" exercises tailor-made for his problems, to perform usually every day. They involve putting joints gently through their full range of motion. This helps maintain normal joint movement, strengthen muscles and helps keep joints in functioning condition so that they can be used the way they are meant to be used.
>
> A proper rest program balanced with a proper exercise program can prevent deformities, and help to correct deformities which have already developed.

Dr. Lawrence Lamb, writing in *Newsday,* says, "It is important to maintain the full range of motion of all joints regardless of the type of arthritis. That is part of the objective of continued exercise."

Mr. Munson always makes it a point to do the special exercises his doctor has given him for his arthritis when his fellow residents at the senior citizens home are participating in my exercise class.

"You keep me at it," he told me. "Everyone needs a little inspiration to keep exercising. My doctor is delighted with the progress I'm making. Even though there's no cure for arthritis, too many people find that the pain of exercising a joint is so severe that they just don't bother, no matter what the doctor recommends. He warned me not to give in, but to put my joints through the gentle motion he's prescribed for short periods each day. That way, he told me, there was a chance that the arthritis might not spread, and that I'd see some improvement. And I have."

If your doctor has given you exercises for arthritis, keep on with them faithfully. Not only are they beneficial for your ailment, but they also improve your general level of fitness.

## The Heart and Muscles

According to the President's Council on Physical Fitness and Sports: "Medical research demonstrates that active persons have fewer heart attacks than sedentary persons. If they do suffer attacks, they recover more readily."

The heart is a muscle, a pump that sends the blood through the body, bringing nutrients and oxygen to all the body's tissues. The heart supplies that energy that makes the other muscles of the body work: the skeletal muscles that enable you to stand and sit, pound a nail into the wall, wash the dishes, dress and feed yourself, walk, get yourself in and out of buses and cars, knit for your grandchildren, work in the garden, drive your car—everything you do that requires movement.

If you don't put your muscles to work, if you allow them to weaken, none of those activities will be easy for you. A visit to a friend will be a chore. The struggle to get into a bus will make you postpone that trip and stay home doing nothing. Your garden will go to weeds. You won't wear that favorite dress because it's gotten too hard to get into it. You'll give up driving before you must. You'll accept aches and pains you never had before, and do nothing to get rid of them.

And the muscle that is your heart will grow weaker along with the muscles in your hands and arms and legs. If you aren't exercising your whole body, you're not exercising your heart, "the engine of life," the most important muscle of all.

We hear a lot about heart ailments these days, and we hear about the respiratory system, circulation of the blood, and blood vessels. We've all seen cases of senility and hardening of the arteries, cases of bones that break and don't heal properly. We've seen our friends and relatives grow older and show signs of age. We've noticed the same thing occurring in ourselves.

But do we really understand that exercise causes the blood to flow more freely, keeps the veins and arteries open, brings nourishment in the form of food and oxygen to all parts of the body, including the brain? Do we understand that like all muscles, the heart can be exercised to stay strong and get stronger? If you use your heart for nothing except to pump blood through an inactive body, how can you expect the heart muscle to remain strong?

The more you exercise, the harder your heart has to work to supply the cells of your body with oxygen and the other muscles with heat and energy. If you do a little exercise that is brisker than a slow walk, you are challenging the heart muscle to work a little harder, and in the process you are making it a little stronger. If you exercise regularly, you will gradually be strengthening your heart. In fact, in preventive and restorative medicine, exercise is deemed so important for the heart that there are now exercise clinics across the United States whose purpose is to strengthen the heart to prevent heart attacks and to restore to health hearts that have suffered attacks.

Finally, the bones that hold our bodies together themselves benefit from exercise. According to Dr. Alexander Leaf of Massachusetts General Hospital and Harvard Medical School, as quoted by Paul Martin in *Parade*, "With lack of activity at any age, our bones lose their calcium salts and become thin and fragile, just as muscles atrophy and become smaller and weaker with disuse. . . . Continued physical exertion remains the most potent measure against this debility."

Exercise, common sense, some understanding of how your body works, and a little will power can equal a healthier, more youthful human being, whatever your age.

## Who Is Old?

What is your age? Fifty, sixty, seventy, eighty, more? Or a lot younger?

Are you old?

I remember clearly an experience I had many years ago. Coming toward me on the street was a boy of sixteen or seventeen. From half a block away, he started to flirt with me. When he got close to me, he took a good look at me and said with complete disgust, "Oh, but you're *old!*"

I was twenty-three at the time.

Measuring age always seems to be done one person at a time, and subjectively.

I said earlier that old age is having your physical impairments rule your life. Old age, too, is in the eye of the beholder. Each of us thinks the other guy is old. Even if he's the same age, we are convinced that we look much younger.

Looking at the wonderful people I teach in my classes, I often find myself wondering, "Just who is old?"

Edie, at eighty-four an ardent participant in my classes, expressed her joy at her agility by saying, "I am so very old, and I feel so very young."

Mrs. Blunt, at seventy-eight, is lively and active, with personality to spare. I saw her weekly at the group exercises, and she always had a smile and a greeting. One day I found Mrs. Blunt in tears. "My boyfriend left me for an older woman," she sobbed.

Mrs. Collins, eighty-three, was brought by her daughter to an old age home to see if she would like to make it her permanent home. It took Mrs. Collins no time to size up her prospective fellow residents, who ranged from sixty to their eighties: "These people are too old for me!"

"Who is old?" asked Mr. Stone. "Not me." At seventy-five, Mr. Stone was just moving out of a retirement home with his newly found sweetheart of seventy to start a new life in his own apartment.

The most touching comment of all is Mr. Bailey's. He's eighty-six, and refers to his eighty-seven-year-old neighbor as "the old man."

Oliver Wendell Holmes said, "To be seventy years young is sometimes more helpful than to be forty years old."

A couple of weeks ago, Mrs. Falk, who is about forty-eight, joined my class for younger adults because her mother shamed her into it. "A year ago," she told me, "my mother at eighty-two was becoming a real problem to the family because of her immobility. We had to do everything for her. Then she upped and joined a senior citizens fitness class at the Y, and today she is a marvel, strong and active and able to walk for miles." Mrs. Falk hung her head. "The truth is, I couldn't keep up with her, so here I am. She made me feel older than she was."

Age is relative; it exists mostly in the eyes and minds of others. You cannot measure it in years alone. What you can measure, though, is how fit you are. The fitter you are physically, the younger you are in mind and body, no matter what your age in years.

Mrs. Milburne is still holding down a job at seventy-four. She lives independently and cares entirely for herself.

"What do I care how old people think I am!" she said one day when I met her on her daily walk. "I have a young body that I exercise. I feel young."

She pointed across the street to a middle-aged woman dragging her feet as she moved along at turtle speed. "What makes that woman thirty years my junior superior to me? I'll match my ability to hers any time."

Then she smiled at me and said, "Just to make it more interesting, I'd give hundred-to-one odds."

I know Mrs. Milburne's stamina, and I wouldn't take those odds.

What is old?

My teenage sons, Mark and David, think anyone over twenty is old. Their parents are well on the way to being ancient. The senior citizens who live next door are too old for words. Yet one day Mark came home from his early morning jogging almost speechless.

"As I was jogging," he told me, "I noticed another jogger about a quarter of a mile behind me on the jogging track. All of a sudden, an old man of about seventy-five caught up with me, and, Mom, he *passed* me! As he overtook me, he said, 'Hello, kid. Goodbye, kid,' and he was a quarter of a mile ahead of me."

Mark went off to school, shaking his head in disbelief—a sixteen-year-old who had had his firm convictions about old age severely shaken.

What is old? It doesn't mean stopping everything you've always done. Just because you reach the magic age of sixty, or whenever old age is supposed to begin, it doesn't mean that a body that has been exercised its whole life suddenly stops working. If you could do fifty pushups the day before your sixtieth birthday, you'll be able to do them the day after, too. You won't *start* doing fifty pushups on your sixtieth birthday if you weren't doing them before, but there are plenty of other things you *can* do.

Old age means that you have allowed your body and its weaknesses to take control of your mind and spirit.

Exercise is not a total answer, but the evidence is so strong that it is an important part of a healthy, vigorous life that you can't afford to ignore its benefits. With it, you can outwalk, out-live, and out-enjoy those who don't exercise. Those other people will be "old." You will be as young as you allow yourself to be.

## THREE

# *Before You Begin*

---

*H*AVE I convinced you that exercise can be a fountain of youth? Are you ready to plunge into a daily routine of exercise and activity?

The answer is—no.

I want you to become fit; I want you to enjoy doing so. I want you to experience the advantages of an exercise program and to understand how much such a program is going to benefit your life. But before you begin, it is absolutely necessary that you understand how to exercise safely, in order to achieve the best that it can give you.

It is, unfortunately, a fact of life that the body is subject to many kinds of ailments and diseases. It docsn't matter what age you are—poor health is not exclusively a condition of the later years. A lifetime program of physical fitness may help prevent some ailments that are common to senior citizens, but some conditions have no proven relationship to a lack of exercise. Whatever your physical condition, however, and whatever your age, there is only one person who can tell you whether or not to begin an exercise program. That person is your doctor.

While I can tell you about the benefits of exercise in general and give plenty of examples of how exercise has helped others, I cannot tell you as an individual whether your physical condition is such that you can undertake an exercise program.

Before you begin, then, have a physical checkup and get an O.K. from your doctor to start a fitness program.

The exercises in this book are designed for older persons with no physical impairment other than those caused by a sedentary life.

The first group of exercises simply suggests ways to get about safely and with ease in your everyday life: sitting, standing, getting in and out of cars, and so forth. They require no special physical exertion, but they are important to you because they show you how to deal with life situations without injury. Those activities are useful for impaired individuals as well as the healthy.

The second group of exercises is especially designed for healthy senior citizens whose bodies are in need of strengthening. It is a basic program which any person without serious physical impairment can undertake. Even if you feel you are in good shape, the sitting and standing exercises in this group are designed to keep every joint and muscle in the body stimulated, and as such, they are essential to maintaining good physical fitness. Even an active senior citizen who is a devoted jogger is not exercising, say, the wrist and finger joints when he runs, so they are a good habit for the well-exercised, as well as for the physical fitness beginner.

The third group of exercises is more challenging. It is designed for older persons who are already in good shape—people who have been exercising regularly over the years. They are also suitable for those who have built up their strength and agility with the sitting and standing exercises in the second group and are ready to add more stimulating exercises to the basic program.

Note that I say *add*. Whatever new exercises you gradually include in your program, don't fail to continue the sitting and standing activities for a well-rounded program.

Before you begin, to decide which group you should start with, consult your doctor. He or she will be able to tell you which exercise will be suitable for you, given your physical condition. If you are in good health, there are no activities in the first and second groups that will harm you. There are no harmful exercises in the third group, provided you are in the proper physical shape.

If your doctor gives you a go-ahead for the basic program, follow the instructions exactly. The exercises have been successfully tested over and over again with senior citizens of all ages. Don't overdo any exercise; follow the directions for the number of times each should be done. If you cannot do the exercises the number of times suggested, do as many as you can, and challenge yourself to work up to the number of times given over a period of days or weeks.

Perhaps your doctor will recommend some form of modified exercise for you. He or she will tell you what kind of program to follow, and what kind of exercise will be most beneficial to you. Of course, if for medical reasons you are advised not to exercise, follow your physician's advice.

## Starting Slowly

A professional football player doesn't go from an easy summer layoff right to the championship game. A person who can barely walk a block without tiring should not expect to go through a series of exercises without fatigue or, in fact, without possible harm to himself or herself in the process. An out-of-condition body cannot be expected to do what a body that has been exercising for years, or even months, can do. The senior citizen needs a program of exercise that will condition the whole body, slowly and gently. This book is written to help you along with your personal exercise program. At the same time, I hope that the activities will help to make your day more enjoyable, and that you will start to look and feel so well that you will think of exercise as one of the most important parts of your day. But you must have patience, and the self-discipline not to force your body to activities for which it is not yet ready.

For example, we are constantly bombarded with advertisements for exercise devices, for spas, for machines that promise us beauty, a better figure, and a magical transformation of our bodies into something perfect. (Seldom do we hear that exercise should be done for health, or for our very survival.)

What the ads do not say is that it is impossible to turn a weak muscle that hasn't been used for years into a strong, healthy muscle overnight. A joint that has lost its flexibility from years of disuse does not become youthful and flexible with a few minutes of exercise now and then.

The temptation is strong to believe the claims we hear, and perhaps to buy a device that asks too much of our bodies. A machine or an exercise device is a convenience, in any event. It may be suitable for a person who knows the capabilities of his or her body. But if you haven't exercised regularly for years, if you are a senior citizen whose aches and pains (and doctor) tell you that you have neglected your body, don't rush out and spend your money on an exercise device.

What about spas? At the health spas that are appearing everywhere, you'll find many of your friends and neighbors, men and women of all ages, in all states of physical fitness. Are you, the senior citizen, ready to join them? Are you ready to be shown a machine that stretches limbs and twists muscles, and jump right in? Remember that most health spas provide only facilities and equipment; they do not provide an understanding of the needs of an older person whose body may be in very poor physical shape. Bones are brittle and muscles are weak. Are you prepared to chain yourself to a machine that may give you muscle fatigue that lasts for weeks? That may break a bone or pull a joint beyond its capability? Are you ready to use a vibrating device which batters the blood vessels? Do you know enough not to rush into a sauna after vigorous exercise, which itself generates heat, but to wait until the body temperature has decreased?

I believe that machines of any sort are crutches. If you sincerely wish to improve your physical state through exercise, you must be willing to do it on your own, proceeding slowly, without relying on any kind of device. The only devices you need are your own mind and your own body. In Chapter Thirteen I will suggest some exercise equipment you can put together from items found in your household; they will make your exercises at home more interesting, but they are not substitutes for your own effort.

A slow start, steady work, and a positive attitude—no excuses —these are what you need to begin and exercise program.

## Attitudes and Excuses

Don't, please, make excuses for not exercising. Don't start and then think up ways to justify your failure to continue.

"Anyhow, my parents never exercised, and they lived to a ripe old age. . . ."

I hear that one every day from senior citizens who are looking for an excuse not to participate in exercise groups. Like you, they are fifty, sixty, and older. They're remembering their parents who lived to eighty or ninety "without a day's sickness." They're thinking that they come from a "long-lived family." There may be such a thing, but I wouldn't sit back and count on living to ninety-five just because my father or mother did.

Did you ever stop to realize how very different life has become in the past thirty years or so? It's far different from the life your parents led, in big ways and small ones. Your parents, fifty or sixty years ago, may not have exercised regularly as we define "exercise" today. But they had to work hard physically all their lives to clean the house, scrub the floors, do the laundry by hand in a big washtub, walk to stores or to a job where much labor was done manually, perhaps plow fields on foot behind a team of horses. Look back on your own childhood and youth, half a century ago, and look at the way young people live now in terms of physical activity. Weren't things a lot different then for you, too?

Each generation before the present one had it harder. They had no pushbutton machines, electrical appliances, cars, trains, whatever makes life simpler today—and less full of physical exertion. So when we say that our parents lived to a ripe old age without exercise, consider what they had to do to live at all: they used their bodies every day and in every way. The same cannot be said of us today. We have to make a special point of exercising our bodies, if we want to reach that same ripe old age.

I firmly believe that one reason women live longer than men is because they are active longer. When a man "retires," it generally means doing nothing, or far less than he did before. A woman has no retirement age. She continues to shop, to cook, to care for the household and her retired husband, just as she has always done. This activity helps keep her in better health and gives her a longer life. This is all the more apparent when an older couple gives up their home and moves into a senior citizens home, where both of them have less to do. Unless the woman maintains her previous activity, she deteriorates as fast as the man.

A friend of mine who has lived abroad in underdeveloped countries remarked that she rarely saw inactive old people there sitting around staring at the four walls. "Everyone, from child to grandmother, was busy doing something all day long to hold life together. It seems, from looking at them, that people who must be busy from birth to death don't suffer from old age."

A young man of my acquaintance, in his thirties, boasted to us one day, "I can't remember a single day when my grandmother was ill. I remember when I was a child, she would run around with us and play our games, giving all of us a good time that none of my friends had from their grandparents."

She had had a very long life, he told us, active until the age of 101, when she injured her back jumping rope!

"She died of an infection after an operation," he said. "Otherwise she probably would have lived another ten years."

"What made her so agile?" I asked him, always eager to find out the secrets that enable older people to live active, vital lives.

"Why, I don't know. She was just like anybody else."

"Wasn't there anything special about the way she lived? Did she exercise?" I persisted in questioning him, and all he could answer was, "No, she never exercised. She was too busy, she didn't have the time."

As the conversation continued about his own life, he mentioned that his grandmother had lived at the top of a steep hill that was practically a mountain.

"I used to have a terrible time climbing that hill," he said. "My grandmother managed to climb it easily five or six times a day, to get back and forth to town and visit neighbors and do her chores."

As he innocently described his breathless climbs and his grandmother going up and down her mountain, I saw at once what had made it possible for her to be jumping rope at the age of 101. The vigorous exercise required to climb a steep hill regularly was enough to keep her body in condition and to enable her to live a long and active life.

Many healthy and agile senior citizens are connected in the same way to an active past, but we are not aware of the connection. And society is not yet ready to credit fully the role of such past exercise in daily living in making an active present possible. We think those active seniors possess some magic formula—or "luck"—that keeps them healthy, whereas it is just a lifetime habit of activity that makes it possible. Some formerly active people, however, find it easier to succumb to the delights of pushbutton living and sitting in an easy chair. They are ignorant of the reasons why they must exercise. Excuses are easier than getting up on their feet.

Laziness is the most common reason for not exercising, whether you are a teenager or a senior. The excuses that come from pure laziness are endless.

"There wasn't a single trick I didn't use so I didn't have to exercise," Mrs. Davis told me. "It was too hot, it was too cold. I was tired, I wasn't feeling well. There was a television program I didn't want to miss. I used every kind of excuse so I wouldn't have to get out of my chair, but the truth was, I was just plain lazy. Then one day my daughter had a serious discussion with me. She wanted to know what nursing home I wanted to go to. Let me tell you, that scared me.

"It got me out of my chair and exercising every day. Instead of going to a nursing home myself, I'm thinking of volunteering at one in our town to help take care of the old people!"

Mrs. Davis, who is now in her seventies, is one of the most active participants in my weekly exercise class.

So put excuses out of your mind. If you want to feel younger, look younger, stay alive longer, and continue to live an independent life, it's going to mean hard work. But it's also going to mean adding enjoyment to your life. You'll find yourself wanting to do more, spend time with people, go about more. Athletes, movie stars, models, people who have to stay fit and beautiful, exercise faithfully. You can achieve fitness and beauty yourself for an independent old age in a healthy body.

## Do's and Don'ts

If you are about to begin an exercise program, there are a few do's and don'ts that you should remember. You want to get the most out of your program, so these few hints will help prevent injury and help you exercise safely and comfortably.

It is never wise to impair your blood circulation at any time, but you should be especially careful when you exercise. Unless your doctor has specifically prescribed a girdle or corset for support, don't wear a girdle when you exercise. Don't wear rubber garters to hold up socks or stockings. Don't wear tight-fitting clothing that might impede circulation. Take off your jacket and tie. Loosen your belt. Keep your body as free of restrictions as possible. Exercise stimulates the blood circulation, so it is unsafe to stop the blood from flowing freely when you exercise.

What kind of clothing should you wear to exercise? Remember that exercise generates heat. When the body is at rest, the muscles generate little heat; during exercise the amount generated increases many hundreds of times. If you are wearing heavy clothing, or clothing made of leather or other materials that keep heat from escaping, it could be harmful. The combination of an increased body temperature and the burden of heavy clothing that doesn't allow the heat to escape or be absorbed can be dangerous.

You should exercise in a cool room wearing light, loose clothing, and preferably no shoes. If you want to take a brisk walk in cool weather, it is advisable to wear a sweatshirt under a lightweight coat rather than a heavy, heat-holding coat. The sweatshirt will absorb the perspiration and the light coat will allow the heat to escape.

You may exercise at any time of the day, except after eating. Eating a heavy meal increases the blood pressure; exercise will raise it even further. When you have just eaten, you have automatically put a little extra stress on the heart, because it must send blood to the digestive system to help it digest the food you have just consumed. If you take a walk or become active immediately after eating, you'll put additional stress on the heart to supply energy to the moving parts of the body along with the digestive system. Of course, after eating, you are likely to feel sluggish and lazy anyhow, and if you are too full to move, you're too full to get the most out of any exercising you do.

Otherwise, you can exercise when you want. Some people feel comfortable with an early morning routine. Others like to have a morning cup of coffee and then get on with their exercises. Some favor the hour before lunch. And many of my class participants like to exercise just before going to bed. They find it relaxing and helpful in getting to sleep at night. (Others, though, find before-bed exercises too stimulating to get to sleep easily. You'll have to decide which kind of person you are.)

Find your individual preference, give yourself an exercise pattern, and stick to it.

Mrs. Berg used to come into my classes feeling completely exhausted. But when she had finished her exercises, she would clench her fist, and with a twinkle in her eye, she would point to the door and say, "Now I can go out and punch this cruel world in the nose!" Mrs. Berg is one of those people who find exercise extremely stimulating!

## The Tennis Player and the Heart Attack

Perhaps nothing illustrates better the need for care in exercising than the tennis player and the heart attack. When someone asks me about the dangers of exercise, the do's and don'ts that everyone should observe, I point to Mr. X. He may be a young man, a middle-aged person, or a senior citizen. He doesn't exercise much—quite likely not at all. He goes to work, he watches television at home. On weekends he putters around the yard. Maybe he and his wife go out to dinner once or twice a week. Mr. X can live in the country, the suburbs, or the city. If he is not yet a senior citizen, he will be in twenty, ten, fifteen, or thirty years.

One day Mr. X decides that it's about time he became active; the propaganda about exercising is beginning to reach him. Perhaps he thinks about jogging—but that means getting up early. How about tennis? His friends are taking up tennis. There's a lot of prestige connected with the tennis club. Or maybe he wants a few hours away from the family. Maybe he remembers enjoying the game when he was younger. Whatever the reason, Mr. X signs up for time on the court and professional instruction. He's going to have half an hour or an hour on Saturday, and he's determined to make the most of it.

His first day on the court, the instructor has him running back and forth, knocking a few balls over the net, trying to return a few serves. He's running, stopping, running, stopping. He's so out of condition that he takes every chance he can get to stop—even if it's just for a second before the instructor sends a ball back over the net to him.

The sporadic running and stopping puts unusual and totally unaccustomed stress on his heart.

Mr. X has a heart attack on the tennis court.

All newcomers to exercise had better keep Mr. X in mind. Exercise, particularly strenuous exercise, cannot be done sporadically, when the exerciser feels like it. Exercise is not something that you can rush into; just as the football player warms up for the football season with training sessions, so must the exerciser warm up his body for a strenuous session of physical activity.

Mr. X probably didn't have a physical examination before he rushed out onto the court. If he had, his doctor would have warned him that vigorous, unaccustomed exercise is unwise without proper conditioning. Mr. X might have understood that his heart might not be able to stand the strain. He observed no safety precautions; he didn't take into account the internal machinery of his body. He didn't understand what exercise is all about. A wise tennis player, and a wise instructor, does not ask his body to endure sudden stops and starts. A wise player knows that motion should be continuous; even when the ball is in the other side of the court, the player keeps moving, so that there is no sudden spurt of activity that puts stress on the heart, followed by complete immobility.

What does that story mean to you, the senior citizen, who is about to undertake an exercise program?

First, of course, you don't exercise unless your doctor agrees that you can.

Second, you must understand how to prepare yourself for exercise so that you do not put your heart and your body under stress that is too great for it to handle. No one should start a program of vigorous exercise, like tennis or jogging, without first conditioning the body through gentle exercise that gradually brings the body to top form. Only then should strenuous exercise be undertaken. And any exercise should follow a pattern of slow beginning (warmup), vigorous exercise within your capability, then a gradual tapering off.

If you are worried about heart attacks and exercise, remember that the chances are greater that you will have a heart attack if you do *not* exercise. That doesn't mean that exercise makes you immune to heart attacks, but exercisers who do have heart attacks have a better chance of surviving them—your heart muscle may be strong enough, because of exercise, to keep going.

## Another Way to Look at Exercise

If the story of Mr. X has made no impression on you, let me give you another way to remember how all exercise should be handled.

An expert lover doesn't rush into things. The expert lover, wooing his sweetheart, starts gently, with great tenderness. He gradually arouses her, warming up the body to a passionate warmth. The lovers reach a peak and then, ever so slowly and gently, the whole act ends in a tension-free and relaxed state of both mind and body.

Exercise is like sex? Yes, and if you can remember that, you will remember how to exercise. Start slowly, gently, to warm up the body. Speed up your activity to stimulate blood circulation, as a lover stimulates his sweetheart. Reach a peak of activity, then taper off with less vigorous motion to bring the body to relaxation.

Keep that expert lover in mind, and you have the key to safe and sensible exercise.

## A Final Safety Precaution

It cannot be said often enough: don't overdo any exercise. Your goal, after so many years of sedentary living, is not becoming Charles Atlas overnight. Be patient with your body. You've waited this long—another few weeks or months will not make any difference. If you are unable to do an exercise as described —if you cannot, for example, lift your foot twelve inches off the floor—don't be discouraged. Lift it as high as you can, even if it is only one inch. Tomorrow, or next week, it may be two inches, then three. With perseverance and patience, you'll make steady progress, and I promise you that you will not be sorry for trying. You will be helping yourself, even if the beginning seems slow.

Mrs. Brown put it aptly not long ago. She stretched out her very steady hands for me to admire, and I recalled when they were weak and trembling.

"I work hard to keep myself in good condition," she said. "It's taken a long time, but these hands would never do anything for me, if I did nothing for them."

# FOUR

# *Life Situations*

$W$HEN I conducted private classes in exercise for people of
all ages, I had a number of senior citizens among my students.
I paid no special attention to them, since they were well-exercised
individuals who kept up with younger class members without
difficulty. In those days, I wasn't aware that for many older people, age is a serious handicap.

I might have remained unaware except for the fact that one
day more than eight years ago, I walked into one of the many
old age homes and hotels in my community that cater to senior
citizens. I did so out of curiosity, and the first person I saw was
an instant education for me. An old lady was just coming out
of an elevator carrying a large pocketbook in her left hand and
a heavy coat over her left arm.

I watched her slowly approach a straight-backed chair with
arms and start to sit. First she put her right hand on the right
arm of the chair, still holding the heavy coat and bag in her
left. Then she put the entire weight of her body on her right

hand, and as I looked on, the woman and the chair toppled to the right. The result: a serious injury for the woman, and for me, a sudden realization of the hazards older people face if they do not understand how to use their bodies. I was determined, then and there, to discover a better way for the aged to perform simple, everyday activities like sitting down in a chair. And I was going to teach as many as I could how to do it.

If you read no further than this chapter, you may save yourself from injury; you will certainly make your life easier. Even if you suffer from medical disabilities that do not allow you to participate in an exercise program, you will learn here how to handle your body so that you are not completely at its mercy and dependent on others for help with your every action.

After witnessing the accident at the old age home, I began studying the physical impairments common to older people in order to develop ways for them to properly sit down, get up, walk, climb stairs, get in and out of cars, and get out of bed. I saw that those skills are necessary for all older people: they are the first step leading to complete physical fitness. Practice these activities as I describe them until they are second nature to you.

## Sitting Down, Getting Up

Common sense is an important ingredient in any activity you perform, whether it is a simple act like sitting in a chair or a strenuous exercise to stimulate the blood circulation. And common sense doesn't stop at sixty, so put it to use as you learn how to manage your body. Remember the old lady who fell when she tried to sit. Common sense tells us that no one should be hampered by heavy parcels on one arm while leaning off-balance on the other.

Los Altos Methodist
Church Library

1. If you are carrying anything—a pocketbook or a package—drop it gently on the floor close to the chair.

2. Stand with your back to the chair. Feel the edge of the chair with the back of your calves. Look to your right and left to make sure that you are directly in the center of the chair. (You must actually *feel* the chair behind you before you sit, or you may end up on the floor.)

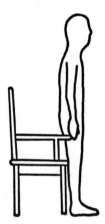

3. With your calves hugging the chair, bring your feet in under the chair as far as you can, with your feet a few inches apart.

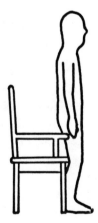

4. Bend your knees, and at the same time, bend your body forward, chin out in front of you. (If you bend your head below heart level, you may get dizzy.) Simultaneously, put your right hand on the right arm of the chair, your left hand on the left arm, and extend buttocks toward the chair.

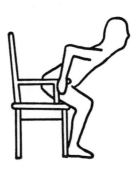

5. Now put all your weight on your hands and lower yourself into the chair.

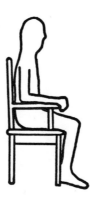

It's a simple and straightforward process, so logical when you understand how it should be done: calves against chair, feet close to it, knees bent, body bent forward, hands on each chair arm, weight on your hands, and you're sitting.

You have learned to sit safely, without chance of injury. Practice that method of sitting every time you do; learn to be conscious of what you are doing with your body.

Once you are sitting down, remember to sit properly. If you slouch in the chair, you can kill your spine, and proper spine alignment while sitting is an important health aid. The buttocks and the shoulders should hug the back of the chair, and the feet should be firmly on the floor.

If you don't own a chair with a firm seat and a straight back, invest in one to give your back and spine a treat—and a rest. When sitting, don't cross your legs, since that impairs blood circulation. If you are short and your feet don't reach the floor, get yourself a footstool so that your feet aren't dangling. Rest your elbows and hands on the arms of the chair.

How about getting up from that same chair? If anything, getting up is harder than sitting down for someone who isn't in good physical condition, but it doesn't have to be a struggle.

1. First, don't try to get up from a chair when you are sitting back in it with shoulders and buttocks touching the chair back.

2. Bring your body forward to the edge of the chair— slide it forward close to the chair's edge, making sure, of course, that you don't fall off. To do that, lift your left thigh and hip and the heel of your left foot, putting your weight on your left toes and right hip. Slide the left hip forward and bring down the left heel. Now do the same with your right hip. Repeat left and right until you have moved your body near the edge of the chair.

3. Bring both feet under the chair, a few inches apart. Bend the body forward at the waist, with your chin pointing forward and up. (Be sure not to bring your head below the level of the heart, as this might make you dizzy.)

4. Put your right hand on the right arm of the chair, your left hand on the left arm. Now put all your weight on

both hands and legs, and bend your body forward as you gently push yourself to a standing position with hands and legs.

When a newcomer joins my classes for senior citizens and starts to sit incorrectly, the others in the class are quick to shout out (sometimes to the newcomer's surprise), "Don't do it!"

The proper method of sitting is the first thing I teach in my senior citizens classes, and I make my students so conscious of right and wrong that they wouldn't dream of doing it any other way. Like you, they have acquaintances who have been injured from falls; and like you, they are sensible enough to understand the importance of what is actually the one activity all older persons must know how to do safely. As we grow older, we spend more time sitting, even in the course of an active life. Knowing how to do it safely is surely one of the most important things we can learn.

## Exercise for Getting Into and Out of Chairs

Your next step is to learn how to stand or sit without the aid of your hands. It is completely unnecessary to lose this ability, and it happens only out of neglect, laziness, or lack of foresight—we don't ever believe that it could happen to us. After working for years with people who have let their bodies go to pot, it still alarms me to see limbs that could have been kept in good condition ceasing to function. For example, because for most people the left hand is not used as much in daily living as the right, and is used even less as we get older and less active, it stops functioning first; the right hand remains in constant use for eating, combing hair, writing, picking up objects. Without steady exercise, the left becomes weak and eventually almost useless.

There is no reason why we cannot work to eliminate problems, or even prevent them from occurring. To that end, I now teach all my older students a simple exercise to be performed daily, to keep the body strong enough to support itself in performing the simple task of getting into and out of a chair without aids—without putting your weight on your hands or using the chair arms. It has worked miracles for senior citizens who have learned how to do it. I am enormously pleased to hear their gasps of surprise the first time they stand up unaided.

1. Stand with your back to the chair, with your calves hugging the center of the seat. Look to see that the chair is directly behind you. Have your feet close to the chair, a few inches apart.

2. Lean your shoulders forward, and at the same time bend your knees *forward* (as opposed to *down*, so the body is lowered), while the buttocks are heading back, toward the chair. Keep your chin pointing outward and up.

3. Keep your hands above the arms of the chair, in case you lose your balance.

4. Now lower your buttocks into the chair from the knees, and sit.

5. Use the same principle to stand, with this variation:

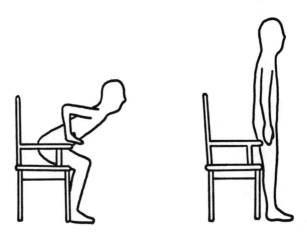

As you are getting up, with your hands above the arms of the chair, bend the body forward, from the waist, pushing out your chest to help propel you up and out of the chair.

6. Repeat this exercise once or twice. If you can do it without difficulty, increase the number of times you perform the exercise, perhaps up to ten times a day or more. If you do have difficulty, don't be discouraged. Keep on trying, and gradually you will get to the point where you can stand and sit easily without resting your weight on your arms. (You will make faster progress when you combine this exercise with the overall fitness program outlined in later chapters.)

## *Up and Down Stairs*

For the physically fit, walking up and down stairs is a marvelous exercise to keep the body conditioned. For the impaired, however, or those who have lost their agility, a flight of stairs can be terrifying. We've all heard stories about people who've fallen on stairs and ended up with broken hips or arms. Many of them are senior citizens who, through lack of exercise, have lost their sense of balance and their agility.

I think of my friend Beatrice, who once lived in fear of the elevator in her apartment building breaking down. "If that happened," she told me, "I'd be trapped. I couldn't manage the one flight of stairs down to the lobby, and I certainly couldn't make it *up* those stairs."

Another friend, Ray, told me that every time he had to go somewhere, he spent the hour before worrying whether he would have to face a flight of stairs when he got where he was going.

Both Beatrice and Ray have learned to condition their bodies through exercise, and stairs no longer hold any terror for them. First I showed them how to eliminate some of the dangers of climbing stairs.

I suggest that anyone who has difficulty with stairs should begin with a short flight (there is no way you can easily turn around in the middle of a long flight and come down if you get tired). The stoop outside a house usually has only three or four steps. It should have a banister or railing, because until you have regained your balance and coordination, you *must* have something to hold onto.

1. Take hold of the banister with the hand nearest it as you stand at the foot of the stairs. Say it is a left-hand banister, which you grasp with your left hand.

2. Bring your left foot up onto the first step.

3. Put pressure on your left hand, which is on the banister, and drag your right foot up and put it on the same step with the left (don't try to lift that right foot—drag it).

4. Step up again, *always* with the foot closer to the banister.

That is the safest way to climb up steps. You are never off-balance.

Coming down stairs, use the same principle.

1. Put your right hand on the banister.

2. Take the first step with your right foot. Make sure the heel of the right foot slides down on the inside (riser) of the step to prevent a misstep and a possible fall.

3. Then bring your left foot down to the same step, again with the heel sliding down along the inside of the step. You will have to rely also on your eyes—just as the strongest and youngest do when walking down stairs—but if you are not careless, you can go up and down stairs easily using this method.

There is no exercise except general conditioning exercises that will enable you to go up and down stairs with no support, but it is a good idea to practice on a short flight of stairs until you unconsciously follow the procedure I have outlined.

## *Into and Out of Cars*

Pauline, who is about eighty-five, was sitting in the lobby of the old age home where she lives when I came by. She was wearing her hat and coat and a big frown.

"Why the long face?" I asked.

"I'm going to the dentist," Pauline replied.

"I don't blame you for looking so sad," I said. "I don't like going to the dentist either."

"Oh, it's not the dentist," she said. "I don't mind the dentist. The problem is that it's such a chore for me to get in and out of the taxi."

We rely so much on cars in this society—to get to work, to do the marketing, and for countless activities during the day. A car represents the means of getting out of the house for a while to visit friends and family. To a senior citizen, particularly if physically impaired, cars may pose a difficulty that can spoil all the enjoyment of going out. Too often, the effort of getting into and out of a car is almost too much.

The principle of getting into a car is the same as sitting down in a chair; getting out is just like getting up from a chair. (I'm talking about sitting in the front seat or the back seat of a four-door car; it is almost impossible for a somewhat impaired person to get into the back seat of a two-door car, and a thoughtful driver will never ask him or her to do so.)

In dealing with cars, the driver has to do his part. He must place the car so that it is easy to enter. Drivers should not bring the car up close to the curb. Many people feel that this will somehow save the senior citizen a few steps, but it is no help at all. It only means that the older person must stand on the curb, which is almost level with the car seat. That requires the body to be lowered from a great height to a sitting position. On the other hand, if the car is parked so that the senior citizen is standing on the street, the distance between backside and seat is much less—it is almost on the same level as the seat instead of high above it.

1. Enter the car from street level, *not the curb*. Never try to get into a car feet-first.

2. Bring your backside to the edge of the seat, with the calves of both legs hugging the side of the seat.

3. Bend your knees while bending forward from the waist as far as possible and pointing the buttocks toward the seat.

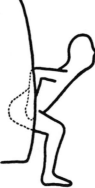

4. Now gently sit down. If your legs are especially weak, you may have to steady yourself with your hands on the door and the back of the seat.

5. Once you are sitting, slide the foot closer to the seat into the car, then bring the other foot in.

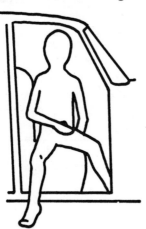
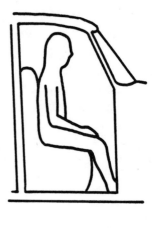

Getting out of a car can be as easy as getting in, and is much like getting out of a chair.

1. When the car door is opened, slide the foot closer to the door out first, then the other foot. With your feet on the ground, or out of the car, edge your body out with the same hip-and-thigh movement used for moving forward in a chair (lift right hip and thigh and heel of right foot, weight on the toes; slide forward on left hip and bring down your foot).

2. When you are near the edge of the seat, bring your feet under you as far as you can, close to the car.

3. Bend the body forward from the waist, keeping your chin up and pushing your chest forward.

4. Put all your strength into your feet and get up. If your legs and feet are not strong enough to do that unaided, put both hands on the car seat and use them to push yourself up.

## Getting Up from Bed

A lot of unnecessary accidents have been caused by sudden blackouts, dizziness, or loss of balance when getting out of bed. Many people don't know how to get up properly after a long rest or a night's sleep. That is not a hazard only for older people; anyone can find himself dizzy and off-balance from leaping up after lying down for a long period.

A middle-aged friend reported her experience not long ago: "I was in a deep sleep when I heard the doorbell ring. Without being fully awake, I jumped out of bed, ran down fourteen steps, and blacked out. I must have been lying there for quite a while, because when I came to, there was no one at the door."

When you are lying down or asleep, the body is completely relaxed, and the heartbeat is at its lowest. Don't, then, jerk your body into sudden action, which demands a more rapid heart rate, by quickly getting to your feet from a horizontal position. Give your body a chance to adjust to a waking, upright position.

1. When you wake up, lie comfortably on your back for a few minutes, with your head raised on a pillow, wiggling your feet.

2. Now sit up slowly, and let your feet dangle over the side of the bed for a minute or two. That brings circulation to your legs.

3. Stand slowly, staying close to the bed in case you feel off-balance; you can sit down again if you feel dizzy.

4. Start walking slowly, increasing your pace only when you are sure that you have your balance and you have no dizziness.

## *How to Sleep*

While we are on the subject of beds and sleeping, there is a sleeping position you might try which is very relaxing. Of course, it's important to have a firm mattress, and I know that it's difficult to change sleeping habits and positions of a lifetime, but try the position whenever you think of it. It puts no strain on any muscles, it takes pressure off the spine, and it doesn't impair circulation.

1. Lie on your side (say, the left side), in a fetal position, with both knees bent toward the chest.

2. Move right knee off the left leg, slightly to the right, placing a pillow under it. That will keep circulation unimpaired.

## Lifting

Even young people frequently injure themselves by lifting objects improperly. The correct way to lift any object is to bend the knees and lower the whole body as far as possible. Then pick up the object with both hands and bring it up with the strength of the feet and the hands. Keep the back straight to eliminate pressure on the spine and back.

However, lifting heavy objects is a strenuous endurance and balancing activity, and I discourage senior citizens from attempting to lift them from floor level. You cannot expect to perform feats of strength that are appropriate only for a laborer, for example, who is accustomed by his profession to lifting from the floor. It is not shameful to admit that there are some things we cannot do, however good our physical condition. Don't hesitate to ask another person to pick up something heavy for you. And don't hesitate to ask, even if it is a light object, if you don't feel able to bend down and pick it up yourself. (There are certain privileges associated with being a senior citizen, and I think that is one of them!)

If you are at home alone and find that bending down to pick up an object is difficult, bring a chair close to the object, sit down as I have described, and *then* pick it up (but remember not to bring the head lower than the heart, to prevent dizziness).

Another simple trick for picking up a small object from the floor is to have on hand a dustpan with a long stick handle. All you have to do is put the dustpan near the object, sweep it into the pan with a broom, and pick up the dustpan.

## Coughing Up Phlegm

The problems that senior citizens face are many; any little tricks that make life easier are welcome. For example, many older persons have difficulty coughing up the phlegm in their throats. Here is an exercise that can help you—and it's also a good exercise to strengthen the throat, neck, and facial muscles.

1. Make believe that you are practicing to enter a contest to see who has the longest tongue. Stick your tongue out as far as you can, pointing it downward toward your chin.

2. Now make a long and loud aaaaah sound, just the way you do when the doctor uses a tongue depressor to look at your throat.

3. Give a healthy cough. Repeat the exercise twice (three times if necessary), and you'll be surprised to see how it helps cough up stubborn phlegm in your throat.

The commonsense approach to all daily activities is especially suited to senior citizens who have not exercised for many years.

No matter what our physical condition, in this modern age we cannot expect to have someone at our side at all times to seat us, to help us up, to get us into and out of cars, into beds, and up the stairs. We *must* be able to manage at least the basic activities of our lives. Senior citizens have a responsibility to care for—and about—themselves. If you are old as you read this, remember that you will be older still. But even though you count your age in decades instead of years or months, you must still strive toward independence, and the miracles that a few minutes of exercise every day can produce.

## FIVE

# *First Exercises:*
# *For Nonbelievers*

---

**Y**ou're just getting older and older sitting there playing cards with your cronies," I chided Mr. Wilson. "You could be getting younger if you'd get up and join the exercise class."

"Exercise is for youngsters," Mr. Wilson replied. "You're not going to get me out there making a fool of myself."

Just as he finished giving me a piece of his mind about exercise, he told his wife to close the door of the rec room at the senior citizens center where he was playing cards. He said he felt chilled.

I immediately challenged him. In front of his friends I bet him that within a few seconds I could make his body feel so warm with a couple of exercises that he'd have to take his jacket off.

"If I lose the bet," I told him, "I'll never ask you to join my fitness class again. But if I win, you have to join in with my other exercisers at the center."

Mr. Wilson agreed, but I could see he didn't believe me. If, like Mr. Wilson, you aren't convinced that your body will really respond to exercise, try this series of one-minute exercises. It will not only make your legs alive and tingly, but also bring flexibility to your knees, loosen up tense muscles in your feet, legs, and thighs, and stimulate blood circulation to bring instant warmth to your whole system.

### *Instant Warmup of Body*

1. Sit straight in a chair (be sure it is steady, and preferably on a skid-proof rug so that it won't slip, but definitely *not* on a slippery floor).

2. Bring your left foot up, with your knee as close to the chest as possible. Put both hands under the knee to hold it up.

3. With as brisk a motion as you can manage, kick your foot forward until the knee is straight, then bring your knee back to your chest. Repeat five times.

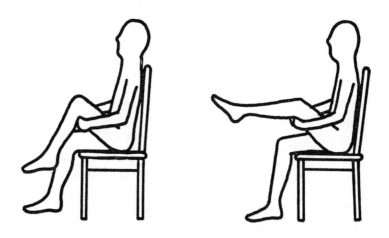

4. Now put your left foot on the floor, and bend over, trying to reach your left ankle with both hands (reach as

far as you can; don't worry if you aren't able to reach your ankle at first).

5. With a brisk motion, massage your left leg upward from the ankle with both hands, especially the calf and the back of the knee. Repeat three times.

6. Stretch your left leg out in front of you, knee slightly bent, and shake the leg as briskly as possible to the count of ten. Put your foot down on the floor. Can you feel the warmth vibrating through your leg?

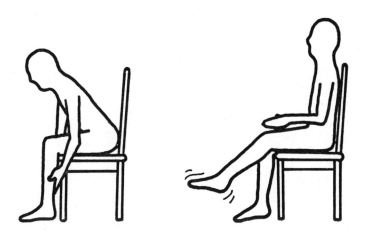

7. Repeat the whole exercise with your right leg.

After one try, Mr. Wilson had to agree that this gentle exercise did make his legs tingle. Then I gave him an exercise for instant warmth that finally convinced him.

Make believe that your body is an old-fashioned water pump, and you are going to pump some water.

1. Sit straight in a chair and stretch your left leg out in front of you, about a foot off the floor (or as high as you can manage).

2. At the same time, raise your left arm in front of you above shoulder level.

3. With an up-and-down pumping motion, bring the foot up and the arm down so that they meet. Move both arm and leg up and down as fast as you can, no more than ten times. (Do this fewer times at first if it tires you.)

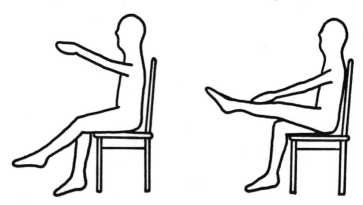

4. Repeat with the right arm and leg.

5. Now raise both legs out in front of you, about a foot apart. Stretch out your arms above shoulder level.

6. Repeat the pumping motion with arms and legs as before, first with the right arm and leg once, then the left once; move right and left alternately to the count of ten. (If you feel tired before you reach the full number, stop at once.)

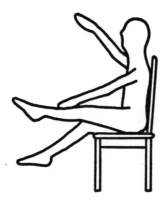

7. Relax, and feel the warmth surging through your whole body.

I won my bet from Mr. Wilson.

"I'm too warm now to keep my jacket on," he agreed, "and I'll try some exercises with the group. But I don't see that the exercise made me a day younger."

One exercise done once won't make anyone younger. No one should expect to regain the vigor of youth in a few minutes. But *minutes a day,* over a period of time, can make all the difference in the world. Exercise is a slow, steady process, but it works.

Norma, who is eighty-two, jokingly offered to split her savings on heating bills with me after I showed her those exercises for warmth.

"I used to get so cold sitting around doing nothing," Norma told me. "Everyone always knew what to get for my birthday— another sweater. And when sweaters didn't keep me from feeling frozen, I'd turn up the thermostat another few degrees. My heating bills got so high that I was going without other things just to pay them.

"But now," she said, "whenever I start to feel cold, I do your instant warming-up exercises, and in no time, I'm taking off sweaters instead of putting them on."

It's much better for you to do some moving around to stimulate blood circulation and warm up your body, than to turn up the thermostat. Too much heat can make you feel sluggish, and the more fuel used to heat your house, apartment, or room, the more it is going to cost you eventually.

## *Walking*

The warming-up exercises are only a beginning—a way for me to demonstrate the power of physical activity, but only a part of an all-around program to condition the entire body. For nonbelievers I also like to point to another exercise that is so obvious and simple, it surprises me so few realize how safe and beneficial it is. I'm talking about walking; it is an ideal way to start yourself moving toward a healthier body.

If there is nothing wrong with your feet, and your doctor tells you that you are perfectly healthy, you should start immediately to increase your walking ability. You don't have to spend your life in an armchair watching television, and you don't have to feel completely exhausted if you walk just a short distance.

We all know how to walk: one foot ahead of the other. But do you know the benefits of regular walking? Walking will improve your health by increasing your stamina, and promoting flexibility of your joints and your general muscle tone. It will make you more agile, and strengthen your heart, blood vessels, and respiratory system. It will help eliminate sluggishness, and make you look and feel better. Most important in one sense, it will make you better able to get about independently, and enjoy a richer, fuller life. A walking program that you stick to helps use up excess calories, so you may lose a few inches in the bargain.

It is important to walk, stand, and sit with the spine properly aligned. Too many of us droop and hunch over for no good reason, and that can make you look older than you are. We don't discipline ourselves to walk properly.

When you walk, stand straight, and pull in your stomach and buttocks. Straighten out your shoulders and hold your head up, but don't tilt it back. Make believe that there is a line up your spine straight through your head.

For a longer and more graceful stride, swing your legs from the hip as you take each step, and let the motion of your hips propel you. Don't walk from the knees; the knee joints are most vulnerable to injury. As you walk, swing your arms freely. Put a bounce in your step.

I have a vivid recollection of walking behind an elderly man who was striding along with a real bounce in his step. When he came to a curb, he literally hopped up or down on it. There was something so jaunty and carefree about him as he proceeded down the street that I speeded up to overtake him. Someone that youthful had to have an interesting story. He was moving along so briskly that I almost had to run after him.

When I was finally able to stop him, he smiled and bowed— and spoke to me in a language I didn't understand.

Then he was off again, with that bouncy step. I was almost glad that his language wasn't one of the several I can communicate in. The picture of that jaunty, joyful old man with his youthful step represented the kind of feeling I have always tried to inspire in the senior citizens I meet in my classes.

## A Walking Program: Where to Walk and When

If you're still adamant against an exercise program, try walking; it will help you get the exercise habit.

Mrs. Avery always found excuses for not joining in my physical fitness group. She couldn't be bothered to exercise at home. She was too tired most of the time to even take walks, or the weather was too bad to go out, or it was another of a hundred reasons. Besides, she kept telling me, nothing was going to do her any good; she was too old (she was not even seventy).

I was determined that Mrs. Avery wasn't going to get away with giving up so easily. I tried reminding her that people who feel physically exhausted all the time without a medical reason need to exercise more than those who don't have that tired feeling.

Finally I said, "Mrs. Avery, I don't want to hear any more excuses about the weather or feeling tired. Your friends are exercising, and so should you. You can walk anywhere—it doesn't have to be outdoors."

This is how I suggested she begin.

Look around the place you live, whether it is a house, an

apartment, or even a room at a senior citizens residence. Choose a route:

> From the living room to the kitchen to the dining room and back to the living room.
> From one end of the living room to the other.
> From one side of the room to the other, back and forth.

Whatever you decide upon, walk the same route over and over again, as many times as you can without fatigue. Keep track of the number of times you can do it. As soon as you feel tired, sit down and relax. An hour or two later, try again. Each time you begin to tire, sit and relax. Try walking your planned route daily, three or four times a day, two or three hours apart.

Each day, increase the number of times you walk your route. Challenge yourself a little, but always remember to listen to your body. As soon as it tells you that you have done enough, sit down—but don't pamper yourself; don't stop for any reason but real fatigue.

If you keep up regular indoor walking, in no time you'll be slowly and gently increasing the number and length of your walks, and you'll notice a definite improvement in your stamina and agility.

Mrs. Avery agreed to follow my suggestions, promising that she would keep to her walking program at home for a while. I also suggested that she turn on her radio to some music and walk in time to that. Someone else suggested she get a pedometer, a gadget that measures how far you walk. Department stores, hardware stores, and sporting goods stores carry them. That way she knew exactly how far she was walking—half a mile, then three quarters, then a mile, all in her own house.

Before long, Mrs. Avery wasn't content with walking in her house. Suddenly she had no hesitation or fear about walking outdoors. First she walked from her house to the grocery store (two blocks), then she was going five, six, seven blocks, and more from her house, and everyone noticed the change in her. She was lively, more youthful, never fatigued.

After she had built up her stamina, I encouraged her to increase her speed, but not the length of her walks. The brisker the walk, the more stimulating it is for the heart and the whole body. Of course, Mrs. Avery noticed the change in herself, too, and went on to an exercise program that conditioned every part of her body (walking alone, for example, does nothing for the flexibility of the joints in the hands).

"I no longer need help to pull me up from a chair," Mrs. Avery said not long ago. "I don't have to look around for someone to walk across the street with, in case I didn't make it before the light changed. All my life I've been praying not for long years but for the strength to be independent of others. But I let myself go, until you showed me how to get back all the strength I'd lost. I was blaming old age for something that was my own fault, and now I've helped my prayers be answered."

Within a few months of starting her walking program, Mrs. Avery, for many years a widow, showed up one day at the senior citizens luncheon holding onto Mr. Graf's arm.

"For years," she announced to the group, "I've been chasing Mr. Graf, but with my old, tired legs, I could never catch him. Now that I have my strength back, I outchased him, and I finally caught him!"

# SIX

# Getting Started on an Exercise Program

*I* have spent most of my life engaged in exercise—for myself and for others. I have seen people crippled by war and disease making a new life for themselves by developing their remaining physical abilities through exercise. I've seen men and women in their eighties and nineties, people who have never exercised, learning how to get up out of their chairs and spend their remaining years as active, alert, and happy human beings. It has given me a great deal of satisfaction to have been instrumental in making that possible. In many cases, the psychological boost that exercise gives is truly valuable. It gives people hope to know that they can reverse the tide and help the body get younger.

I know the powers of exercise first-hand, not only through seeing senior citizens in my various classes begin new lives, but personally. When I was a teenager, I lost my left hand and part of my left arm in a concentration camp in Germany. After only months of not using that arm, the diameter of the limb dwindled to that of my thumb. When I eventually ended up in a hospital, I was referred to physical therapy, and through exercise the muscles in that arm were rebuilt to normal. If the arm had been left unattended and unexercised, the muscles of my whole left side could have atrophied, through lack of exercise.

I have proof, in my own life, of the miracles that exercise can perform. I have seen a great many successes in others, with perseverance and determination. Nothing was accomplished overnight; it wasn't a case of a couple of exercises now and then, when the person was in the mood. It was slow, steady work, but it was worthwhile. It was work those people believed in. They followed a program of nonstrenuous but steady exercise, day in and day out. As I worked with them, I tried to make what they were doing meaningful and enjoyable, reminding them of the important goals they were working for: independence, health, a sense of well-being.

All that is possible for you. In the following pages I will outline an exercise program that is suitable for older persons who have their doctors' approval to undertake exercise.

You must get yourself into the habit of doing exercises every day—at nine in the morning or at eleven just before lunch, at three in the afternoon or just before going to bed. If you establish a pattern of daily exercise at the same time, you will soon find that if you miss it for just one day, your body will notice it.

I've talked about the value of walking, and I've made suggestions on how to map out an indoor route at home. This means that you can walk a planned route every day, regardless of the weather, and can build up strength so that you can include outdoor walks without fear of fatigue—you will have learned your walking capacity. I've suggested that you practice climbing stairs, starting first with a short flight, such as those at the front or back doors, which are usually no more than three or four steps. The exercise for sitting in a chair without the aid of your hands is important for anyone who wants to keep the body from becoming his or her master.

## *Balance and Coordination*

Many older people suffer from a lack of coordination and balance. The physical fitness program presented in this book is designed to increase balance. The fitter your body is, the fewer your balance and coordination problems will be. However, here are specific activities to help those problems.

1. Place a piece of string about four or five feet long on the floor in a straight line.

2. Try walking the string, putting one foot in front of the other, to test your sense of balance.

3. If you have difficulty walking the line, do this easy exercise several times a day. (If you normally use a cane as an aid for walking, start off with it, but hold the cane up if possible. It is there if you need it for support, but you may soon discover that it isn't as necessary as you thought.)

Here is a good exercise to do if you have grandchildren whom you want to spend time with.

1. Get yourself a rubber ball, four inches or more in diameter.

2. Line up a willing grandchild and toss the ball back and forth. It will work wonders for your coordination.

3. If you have no one to throw the ball to, get three or four balls and a wastebasket. Put the basket five feet or so from a chair and try tossing the balls in. If you can do it from five feet, move the basket farther away.

4. Do this exercise two or three times a day, moving the basket farther away as your aim improves.

## *Posture*

"I never once realized all those years," Mrs. Greene said, "that nothing was going to help me when I walked out of the beauty parlor every Friday with a head like Zsa Zsa Gabor's and the posture of the Hunchback of Notre Dame. It was only after I started exercising and being conscious of my posture—and started getting compliments on how well I looked—that I realized I was straighter and taller than I'd been for years. I *felt* like Zsa Zsa!"

Bad posture, a hunched-over body, is not a symptom of old age. It's a bad habit. Maybe it's a lack of awareness, too; we can't see ourselves as others do, looking old and tired.

There's no reason why anyone has to droop. If you do, you've probably neglected to exercise and keep your muscles in proper tone. You're guilty of letting the muscles of your body shrink and weaken instead of keeping them firm and strong. Those weak muscles pull down every part of the body, and the result is a droopy, old-looking person.

Martha came to my classes hunched over, and seemingly unable to straighten up. "Nothing will help me," she said. "I've been hunched over for as long as I can remember."

Exercising diligently for seven months, Martha did straighten out her shoulders. As a result, she found relief from the backaches from which she had suffered for years, and her posture improved 100 percent.

"I just got a compliment," Martha told me one day after an exercise session. "My cousin, who hadn't seen me in a year, couldn't get over how well I looked. He kept on saying, 'Martha, there's something different about you. What is it?' Then he burst out with, 'Martha, you rascal, you've gotten taller!' "

It's not too late to start learning to stand up straight.

1.  Stand straight, with your shoulders back. Pull in your stomach and buttocks.

2.  Keep your head high but not tilted back, remembering that straight line that runs from your head through your spine. (Keeping your head high also helps prevent a double chin.)

3.  To test your posture, stand with your back to a wall, with both heels a few inches from the wall and your hips, shoulders, and head touching it. Walk away from the wall. That is correct posture; practice it whenever you walk.

Remember to sit properly, with shoulders and buttocks against the back of the chair (and avoid soft, overstuffed chairs, which are luxuries our spines can't afford).

Awareness is important. Be aware of your posture while you are sitting, standing, or walking. It does no good to make a joint flexible, or a muscle strong, if you defeat the purpose of exercise by slouching and drooping for the remaining hours of the day.

## Your Capacity for Exercise

Everyone has a different capacity for exercise. No standard applies to all of us. The daily minimum that is right for you must be measured by your physical capabilities, the point at which you reach exhaustion, your rate of breathing, and your pulse rate.

The simplest way to determine your capacity for exercise is to judge when you start breathing heavily after an exercise like walking. If it takes only minutes to make you breathe hard, your capacity is low, so when you begin doing exercises, you should limit yourself to only a few minutes a day.

For both muscle-toning and flexibility exercises, you will have to discover what your capacity is. It's dangerous, for example, to overdo muscle-toning exercises. You could be bedridden for weeks if you don't follow directions and listen to your body. A muscle that hasn't been used for years is *sick,* and unless you treat it with loving care, as you try to get it back into shape, the result could be serious.

An unused muscle *can* be brought back to life, even after years of disuse. It needs to be used steadily and slowly, however, to bring it back to health.

Start by working each set of muscles for no longer than two minutes a day for the first few weeks. Muscles don't hurt while you are exercising them. The reaction to waking up those tired muscles and putting them to work usually comes the day after you start. That's when you might feel some aches and pains. But you'll be defeating your purpose, and possibly harming yourself, if you overdo your exercises the first weeks of a program. Don't let enthusiasm run away with you. There's nothing to be gained from a day's strenuous exercise followed by three days in bed to recover.

Start off with a few minutes of exercise, and then wait until the next day to see your body's reaction to the workout. If you have no reaction—no sore muscles or stiffness—go ahead with the groups of exercises outlined in later chapters, extending your time by a minute for each one. Each day tone the muscles and exercise your joints a little longer, judging how much you can do by your body's reaction the next day. If you are very stiff and sore, don't increase your time, but don't be too easy on yourself.

You can never go wrong by starting off very slowly and paying attention to your body's signals. Of course, if at any time during exercise you find that it is painful or exhausting, sit down and relax. You have probably reached your limit, and if there is much pain, you should see your doctor. However, don't expect exercise to be "painless." Muscles that haven't been worked for years are going to protest a little. Remember too that you are exercising your will power—the will to exercise—and sometimes exercising the will power can be painful, too!

# SEVEN

# *Breathing*

---

$A$NY exercise we do increases the body's need for oxygen. When we exert ourselves, our breathing rate increases to meet the body's demand for oxygen. It is natural, on such occasions, to breathe faster or more deeply. Our breathing mechanism automatically adjusts to the needs of the body, and so I believe that our breathing habits should not be tampered with in general.

I asked one of my athletic sons what he could think of to say about breathing, hoping he had some youthful insight I was not aware of.

He looked at me seriously for a moment and said slowly, "Breathe in, breathe out. Breathe in, breathe out."

My son was right; you breathe in and out, and according to your needs, you breathe faster or slower. However, while doing the exercises described in the book, you will have to take some deep breaths to replenish oxygen and to relax the body. Although while doing strenuous exercise the automatic breathing system takes over, during slower exercises, you can control your breathing to your advantage, and exhale and inhale deeply and rhythmically, without, of course, holding your breath.

## Breathing Safely

Take a deep breath through the nose, while bringing the shoulders back. Blow it out through your mouth while collapsing your shoulders. Don't hold your breath at any time. Some people find it relaxing to breathe in deeply through the nose, then exhale the same way.

Repeat that form of breathing only twice at one time. You might practice it a few times during the day, and you will often breathe this way during exercise.

At an exercise session, one of my students asked, "How are you supposed to breathe when you're jogging or walking fast?"

My answer was, when your body demands oxygen, you don't stop to think how you are going to breathe. Again, you breathe in, breathe out, at the rate your system requires.

Ever since I can remember, so-called experts have been telling me how to breathe effectively. Everyone was an authority. My tailor who lets out the seams on my skirts seemed to feel that if I contracted my stomach muscles when I inhaled, it would make my clothes fit better. In the Army they tell you to throw out your chest and breathe. Yogis think they have invented the perfect way of breathing. They teach you to inhale while inflating your stomach and exhale while you deflate it. This happens to be the correct and natural way to breathe, but not because yogis or anybody else invented it. Experience it for yourself. When you are in bed and relaxed, notice how your breathing becomes deep and rhythmic. You will automatically inhale deeply and inflate your stomach; it deflates as you exhale.

## Yoga Breathing

Don't experiment with yoga breathing. The only place for it is in well-supervised yoga classes under an experienced teacher.

Even then I have witnessed too many unpleasant happenings after yoga breathing sessions, including dizziness, fainting, and vomiting. In my own experience, I have felt extremely uncomfortable after holding my breath for a while, even though I have studied yoga. Since our breathing mechanism has served well so far, the senior citizen should not attempt to change the breathing habits of a lifetime.

Dr. Lawrence Lamb wrote in *Newsday,* "Deep breath holding can set off irregularities in the heart. . . . It can also cause the heart to stop temporarily. . . . Breath holding after deep breathing is particularly bad. I have seen a heart stopped longer than twelve seconds in a healthy subject with this maneuver."

## *Breathing in Cold Weather*

Many of us associate deep breathing with being out in the fresh air, especially in the sharp, clear air of winter. Some of my students boast of opening up their windows on cold winter mornings and sticking their heads out to breathe the cold air. I always discourage that practice as dangerous. Have you ever walked outdoors on a cold morning and found that you couldn't catch your breath? You probably had to cover your nose and mouth with a scarf to warm up the air you were breathing. The same thing is happening when you stick your head out the window.

If you want to get some of that fresh air when you get up, open the window and let some air into the room to warm it up a little. Then take your deep breaths.

When exercising outdoors in cold weather, remember that the air you're breathing should be warmed up, too. Also, exercise causes you to breathe more vigorously and deeply, so some sort of protection is doubly necessary for the nose and mouth. A light scarf over them will help warm up the air you breathe as you exercise or walk outdoors.

I don't advise outdoor exercise in very cold weather, but if you don't want to break a regular exercise habit such as walking, there is a special face mask on the market which is worn over the nose and mouth and which helps warm up the air you breathe to a comfortable temperature.

## Breathing in Hot Weather and High Pollution

It can be dangerous to exercise heavily in very hot weather, when your body may demand too much oxygen, more than the breathing mechanism can supply without strain. Also, since exercise generates heat, in hot weather you may tax the heart and respiratory system beyond its endurance. So, in very hot weather, take walks early in the morning, late in the afternoon, and in the shade. Do gentler forms of exercise that don't demand too much exertion.

If the pollution level is high, try not to do any strenuous exercises outdoors so that you don't breathe in any more polluted air then necessary. Certain types of masks are also on the market for high-pollution areas, but even with those, I don't suggest you exert yourself outdoors.

Remember to allow your body to control the rate of breathing according to its needs. Take a couple of deep breaths between each exercise according to the instructions at the beginning of this chapter, but beyond observing reasonable precautions during extremes of temperature, let your body supply its own needs.

# EIGHT

# Basic Program: Chair Exercises

---

**W**HETHER you are chairbound or able to move freely, the exercises in this chapter are a must to keep all your joints in good working condition. Even if you are already a regular exerciser (say, a jogger or tennis player), these exercises are essential to keep all your joints and muscles in good shape, even the ones you *don't* use on the jogging track or tennis court.

If the instructions specify lifting a limb to a certain height, and you can do it, fine. But if you cannot, do what you can. If I tell you to lift your leg a foot off the floor and you can only manage an inch, that inch is tremendously important. With practice and determination, it will soon be two inches, then three. You'll notice a vast improvement each time you exercise.

In these chair exercises, observe the following practices. Sit in a straight, steady chair with a firm seat. Be sure that the legs of the chair are on a nonskid surface, and that the chair itself is heavy enough so that it won't tip over easily.

I can't urge often enough that both beginning exercisers and well-conditioned older persons should include these exercises in their daily routine. The former should consider them the first step in a program that eventually should include more strenuous activities; for the latter, they are a means of keeping all areas of the body in top condition.

## Legs, Spine, Shoulders, Torso

*To strengthen and loosen up joints in legs and thighs:*

1. Sit straight in a chair. Stretch the right leg out in front of you, an inch or so off the floor.

2. Move the foot around in a circular motion from the ankle. Repeat five times in each direction. Repeat with the left foot.

1. Lift your right leg up about three feet off the floor (or as high as you are able), with knees straight as possible, toes pointing forward.

2. Turn the whole foot, leg, and thigh all the way to the right, hold to the count of five.

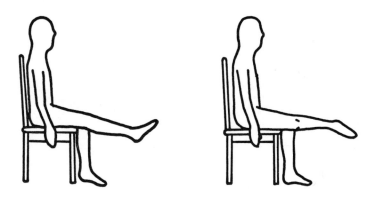

3. Now turn the leg all the way to the left and hold to the count of five. Repeat five times each way. Repeat with the left leg.

*To loosen up kneecaps, thighs, and buttocks:*

 1. Sit straight in a chair, with shoulders relaxed. Bring the left knee up and all the way into the chest, with the aid of your hands if necessary.

 2. Stretch the leg all the way out in front of you in slow motion, with the knee as straight as possible and then lower the leg to the floor, also in slow motion. Repeat five times. Repeat with the right leg.

*To loosen up the spine and midsection:*

 1. Pretend that the chair you are sitting in is a rocking chair.

 2. Rock the body forward and backward very gently. Repeat ten times.

*To strengthen rib cage and relax shoulder muscles:*

The combination of these motions is especially helpful for individuals who have lost the ability to raise their arms—for example, to perform such simple activities as combing the hair.

 1. Put your right and left hand together in an interlocking position.

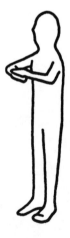 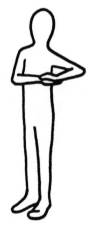

2. Without moving your body, bring the interlocked hands as far to the right as you can, then as far to the left as you can. Repeat five times to each side.

3. With your hands still interlocked, bring them out in front of you as far as you can, and slowly lift them upwards, bringing them to the back of your head.

4. With the arms still interlocked, lower them from the raised position to below your chest. Raise and lower arms five times.

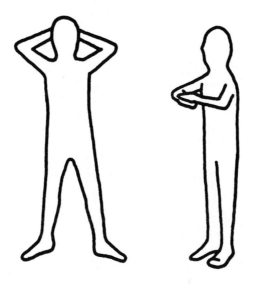

*To loosen up shoulder blades:*

1. Touch your right shoulder with the fingertips of your right hand.

2. With a circular motion, move the right elbow around and around, moving from the shoulder. Repeat five times. Repeat with the left shoulder.

*To loosen the hip joints:*

1. Bring the buttocks forward while your shoulders hug the back of the chair. Hold the back legs of the chair (near the seat) with both hands for balance.

2. Lift the right leg as high as you can, and with a circular motion, move the whole leg in a circle, from the hip. Make five circles, then repeat with left leg.

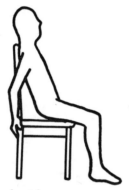 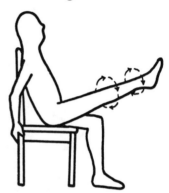

*To stretch sides:*

1. Sit straight in the chair, with knees a few inches apart for balance.

2. Bring your right hand down to the floor (or as far as you can), while raising the left arm as high as you can, with the hand reaching toward the ceiling.

3. Bring the left hand down to the floor, and raise the right arm. Repeat five times with each arm.

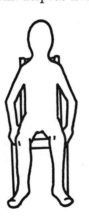 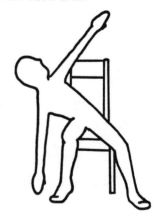

*To stretch the spine:*
Maude Marks came into my exercise class one day apologizing for being so late.

"The podiatrist was at the hotel today," she said, "and he delayed me."

When I remarked that it was too bad she was having trouble with her feet, she said, "Oh, my feet are fine. The podiatrist just cuts my toenails—I can't bend over to do it myself."

I immediately gave Mrs. Marks some exercises for the spine, and explained how important it is to keep the spine healthy and flexible, and not just for reaching down to cut toenails.

The spine supports the body: it also covers and protects the spinal cord, the nerve center of the body, which is connected with the brain. Each vertebra that makes up the spine must be kept flexible, like every other joint of the body. Otherwise the spine becomes stiff and immobile; bending is difficult or impossible, as are movements of the torso in other directions.

In doing this spine exercise, rather than bringing your head down as you bend your body, point your chin out in front of you. Look out in front of you rather than down at the floor. This will help prevent dizziness.

1. Sit straight in your chair. Stretch both legs out in front of you.

2. Stretch both hands out in front of you, parallel to your legs.

3. Bending forward, try to touch your toes with your hands. (Don't worry if you can't touch them at first; come as close as you are able without straining.) Sit up. Repeat five times.

*To permit total movement and stimulation of the body:*

1. Sit straight in your chair, with your buttocks all the way back, touching the back of the chair. Hold your hands up in front of you, elbows bent and pointing outward.

2. Using your entire body (shoulders, elbows, torso, hips, buttocks, thighs), move your body forward to the edge of the chair. Use the shoulders and elbows to propel you forward as you slide the right, then the left, buttock forward. (Be careful not to fall off the edge of the chair.)

3. When you reach the edge of the chair, use the same motion to propel yourself backward to your original position. Repeat the exercise as many times as is comfortable.

## Hands, Fingers, Wrists, Elbows

Our hands, fingers, wrists, and elbows must be given very special care if we are to continue to use them fully as we grow older. Remember how the hand that is used for eating, writing, and other daily tasks has a way of surviving better than the other.

The following exercises are designed to keep hands in good working condition. They are simple, and you need no aids to do them, so you can do them anywhere, anytime, sitting down alone or with friends, or even standing. Your hands may get tired if you do all the exercises given in succession, or if you try to do them too many times at once. I suggest you don't repeat any move more than once. It is always a good idea to rest between exercises if you feel fatigued. At the end of each hand exercise, shake the hands briskly and massage them to relax the muscles and bring circulation to the hand area. Some of these exercises are isometric. Do them with care, and never go beyond the count given. (See Chapter Twelve.)

*To flex fingers and hands:*

1. Flex the fingers of both hands at once by opening and closing them as fast as you can. Repeat about ten times. (This is a good exercise to do anytime you're not doing anything else with your hands.) Let hands hang loose at the wrist, shake briskly, and massage.

2. Flex the fingers of both hands so that the fingers touch the thumb—make a bird's beak. Press the fingers to the thumb, with the thumb resisting the pressure. Hold to the count of five.

3. Stretch both hands out in front of you and separate the fingers as wide as possible (really stretch them apart). Hold to the count of five.

4. Alternate Steps 2 and 3 so that you are first pressing the fingers together, then spreading them apart. Repeat five times. Then relax, shake hands from the wrist, massage briskly.

*To aid muscle toning, flexibility, circulation for hands and fingers:*

1. Stretch out your hands, palms down, keeping your elbows as straight as possible.

2. Make believe you have just found a precious jewel. Make a tight fist and clutch the jewel as if someone were trying to take it away from you. Hold to the count of five.

3. Now throw the jewel away. Let your hands go limp and shake them briskly from the wrist. Massage one hand with the other.

1. Stretch both hands out in front of you, palms down, with your fingers pointing forward.

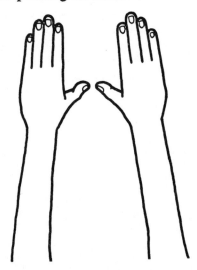

2. Spread your fingers apart and very slowly turn the hands inward to a palms-up position, keeping the elbows straight if possible. (Feel the muscles toning in your hands and all the way down your arms.)

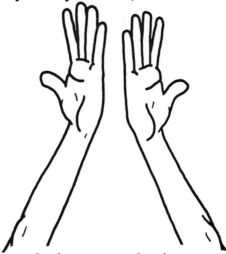

3. Now, very slowly, turn your hands over to the palms-up position. Hold to the count of five. Let your hands go limp, shake, and massage.

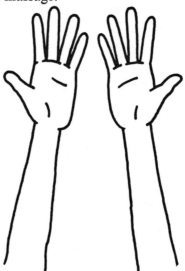

*To strengthen wrists:*

An accident from falling means that senior citizens often end up with broken wrists, because they use their hands instinctively to break a fall. Broken wrists often leave hands completely disabled, so these wrist-strengthening exercises are important.

1. Stretch both hands out in front of you, palms down.
2. Flip both hands down from the wrist, fingers pointing toward floor. Hold to the count of five.
3. Bend both hands up from the wrist (toward the ceiling, and preferably back toward the arm). Hold to the count of five. Repeat five times, using a rhythmic motion.

1. Press right pinky against right thumb, left pinky against left thumb, leaving the other fingers loose.
2. Flex the elbow slightly inward, and flip the hands briskly to the right and then the left from the wrist. Repeat five times.

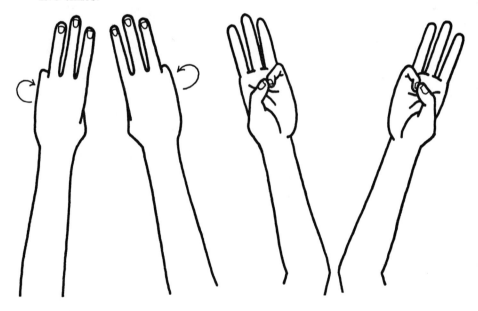

*To promote elbow flexibility:*
Many senior citizens walk around with their elbow joints completely locked from years of nonuse. To help prevent this from happening to you, or to regain the flexibility you may have lost, try the following exercises.

1. Stretch both hands out in front of you, palms up.
2. Touch your shoulders with the tips of your fingers, bending your elbows outward.
3. With a rhythmic motion, stretch your arms out, then bring the hands back to your shoulders. Repeat five times.

1. Stretch both hands out in front of you, palms down.
2. Touch the right hand to the left elbow and bring it back to position. Repeat with left hand and right elbow.
3. With a rhythmic motion, alternate right and left hands, repeating five times for each hand.

In doing these exercises for the legs, torso, hands, elbows, and wrists, don't worry if you can't at first do all of them as many times as suggested. Take your time at the beginning. If you do them regularly every day, you'll find that your joints will get more and more flexible. Soon you'll be able to perform the exercises the suggested number of times.

# NINE

# Basic Program: Standing Exercises

$A$ s we get older and have less to do, it's natural just to take it easy and lounge around, watch our favorite TV programs in a comfortable chair, read a magazine or book, play cards. The fact is, the easy chair is not our best friend but one of our worst enemies—if we let ourselves become dependent on it. Don't let it happen; for any excuse at all, get out of that chair and give your body a chance to work a little. In doing so, you'll improve the body's functions and probably enjoy yourself more, too.

Just as in the case of sitting exercises, observe a few precautions. Take off your shoes and stockings when doing standing exercises. That gives you better balance, and also frees the feet for better circulation. It is advisable to stand behind a chair so that you can use the back for support if you lose your balance.

In the beginning do each of the standing exercises twice rather than doing one of the exercises ten times, which will tire you out before you've worked on every part of the body. If you repeat all the exercises daily, doing them twice each for the first few weeks, your body will grow accustomed to them, and you'll be able to increase the number of times you can do each one. Of course, if you are already in good physical condition and are including the standing exercises as part of your overall fitness program, you should be able to start off doing them without difficulty.

If you feel dizzy or tired the first few times you do these exercises, stop at once, relax, and try again in a couple of hours. But don't give up.

Rhythmic exercises are the safest ones to do, since sudden jerking of any part of the body may cause a pulled muscle or other discomfort. With slow, rhythmic exercises, the danger is lessened. There is less chance of making a sudden move that might pull a muscle, and if you should feel any discomfort, you can stop immediately.

There are many different exercises to choose from, but the nine basic moves given here are designed to touch every part of the body. Here and throughout the exercises in this book, I often have you alternate different parts of the body—say, shoulders, knees, fingers, and back to shoulders again. That keeps you from putting too much strain on one part of the body for too long a time. If a limb has not been exercised regularly for years, it is vulnerable to fatigue. Alternating different parts of the body also helps keep the exercises from becoming monotonous.

*Warmup:*
It is always safest, before you start using your body for any exercise, to begin with a warmup that gradually prepares the body for more vigorous activity.

    1. Start off with a little walk around the room.
    2. Walk for about five minutes or so, increasing your speed. That promotes flexibility of the joints, loosens up

stiff muscles, increases the body temperature and heart rate, and prepares the body for more fatiguing exercises.

*Loosening up spine:*

1. Stand straight, feet shoulder-width apart, hands on hips.

2. With a gentle, rhythmic motion, bend the body forward from the waist, return to an upright position, and bend backward from the waist, bringing the shoulders back slightly. Don't tilt your head back, since you might lose your balance or get dizzy. Repeat five times.

*Shoulder conditioner:*

1. Stand straight. Stretch both hands out in front of you, palms down, with elbows as straight as possible.

2. Bend your elbows and bring them back behind you, as if you wanted your shoulder blades to meet. Hold to the count of five. Repeat five times.

*Loosening kneecaps:*

1. Stand straight, feet shoulder-width apart, and with your hands stretched out in front of you for balance.

2. Bend your knees slightly and straighten up with a bouncing motion. Repeat five times.

*Waist and torso:*

1. Stand straight, feet shoulder-width apart for balance, your hands on your hips.

2. With a rhythmic motion, twist the body to the right at the waist, come back to position, twist to the left, and back. Repeat five times.

*Stretching:*

1. Stand straight, feet shoulder-width apart. Raise both hands above your head.

2. With the right hand, reach for the ceiling as if you wanted to grow a little, and feel the stretch on your right side from the hip upward.

3. Relax your right hand, but keep it raised above your head, and repeat the stretching motion with your left hand. Repeat five times with each hand.

4. Finally, stretch both hands toward ceiling, hold to the count of three, and relax before the next exercise.

*Spine exercise:*

1. Stand straight, knees slightly bent, with your shoulders bent forward slightly.

2. With a rhythmic motion, using both hands, bend to touch your knees, your shins, your toes (if you can), then back to the shins, the knees, and straighten up. Repeat five times.

*Shoulders and elbows:*

1. Stand straight, feet shoulder-width apart, with your arms stretched out at your sides at shoulder level, palms up.

2. With a rhythmic motion, bend the right elbow and touch the top of your head with your right hand. Swing the right arm back to position, and repeat with left hand. Alternate right and left hands, five times for each.

*Standing exercise with a chair:*

1. Stand behind a chair, making sure that it is steady and that you are properly balanced. Hold onto the back of the chair with both hands.

2. Lift your left knee up and bring it in toward your chest (lift it as high as you can), then stretch your left leg all the way out behind you. Repeat five times, then repeat the whole exercise with your right leg. (See next page.)

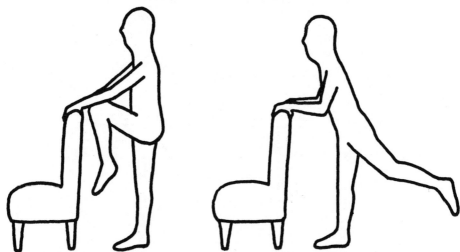

These nine standing exercises, together with the sitting exercises in the previous chapter, should make up your basic daily exercise program, together with regular walking.

## TEN

# Special Exercises: Neck, Tension, Sleep

$M$RS. Miller at sixty-seven wanted to start a new life and acquire new freedom by learning how to drive. She made arrangements to take lessons from a driving instructor, but when the day came, the first time she had to turn her head to see traffic as she pulled from a parking space, she couldn't do it. Her head wouldn't turn sufficiently, and she gave up on the spot, a failure before she had even begun.

"My neck was so stiff," she told me later, "I couldn't turn it at all. My doctor couldn't help me. He said there wasn't a thing wrong with me. I guess he thought that a stiff neck was just one of the symptoms of growing older."

One day, shortly after her failure in the driver's seat, Mrs. Miller wandered into an exercise class I was holding, and got interested. After class she asked me if there was anything she could do about her stiff neck. There was. We worked together for three months, and it changed her life. Back to the driving instructor, and this time she learned to drive with ease—her neck was now as flexible as a woman half her age.

"I'm so grateful for my new freedom," she told me while

proudly displaying her new driver's license. "Driving has made me the most popular woman in town. And," she added, "it sure beats being cooped up by my four walls."

How many times have you seen friends and acquaintances turn their whole bodies around to acknowledge a greeting or to speak to someone behind them? Do you, perhaps, do the same thing yourself without being aware of it? Neck muscles are possibly the least exercised muscles in the body during the course of our lives. An inflexible neck in a senior citizen gives an immediate impression of old age, more than almost anything else.

Closely related to unexercised neck muscles are tension headaches. The U.S. Department of Health, Education, and Welfare, in a study called "Headache: Hope Through Research," says:

> Undoubtedly the commonest of chronic headaches is the muscle contraction headache which comes from stiffly set muscles in the neck. A popular name is "tension headache." . . . The pain can be mild or more severe than some "dangerous" headaches.

Mrs. DiCara, another of my students in the senior citizens exercise class, used to suffer frequently from tension headaches before I began working with her.

"In those days," she said, "there was no relief for me. I was blinded by headaches, and nobody could tell me anything except that they came from 'tension.'"

Exercise itself is of great value in relieving tension in the whole body, but there are also specific exercises for the neck that can bring flexibility and loosen up the tense muscles that cause these headaches.

"I can't believe my days of suffering are gone forever," Mrs. DiCara said recently. "Now, if I feel a headache starting, I do the exercises I learned from you, and it's almost miraculous how the ache eases away."

If you suffer from tension headaches and your doctor cannot

find anything medically wrong with you, or if you have a chronic stiff neck that hampers your movements, try the following exercises to bring relief. Because of the danger of injuring your neck if you don't do the exercises properly, remember always to move very gently. A slow, lazy motion is best. To avoid pulled muscles, don't force your movements or jerk your neck. When you exercise your neck and tension disappears, you may feel dizzy or so relaxed that you will want to close your eyes and doze. For that reason, you should never do neck exercises standing up. Sit in a chair with your body relaxed, your feet on the floor or a footstool, and your hands in your lap.

### *Neck and Tension Exercises*

*Neck exercises:*

    1. Sit in a chair. With very slow, molasses-like motions, let your head fall forward so that the chin rests on the chest. You can feel the pull in the back of your neck. Hold for a slow count of five.

    2. Very slowly lift your head up and let it fall all the way back, so that the back of your head presses into the vertebrae at the base of your skull. (The vertebrae may be stiff and tense from lack of exercise, so this action may cause some discomfort at first.) Hold for a slow count of five. Repeat the forward and backward motions twice.

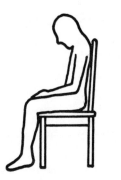 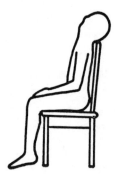

3. Very gently turn your head to the right, pointing your chin at the right shoulder. Feel the pull on the left side of your neck. Hold for the count of five. Very slowly face forward again and repeat to the left side. Repeat twice to each side.

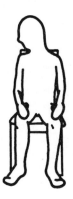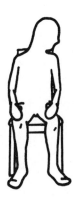

4. Locate the vertebrae at the base of your skull with your hand. Gently massage the vertebrae with a firm, circular motion, at the same time rocking your head back and forth. Repeat five times.

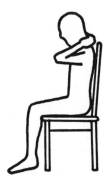

5. Let your head fall forward lazily, and with a circular motion, move it to the right, up, to the back, left, down. Reverse and repeat three times each way.

By this time, you will feel so relaxed and drowsy that you may start yawning. Don't break the magic feeling of relaxation. Instead, close your eyes, let your chin drop to your chest, and relax the whole body. Stay in that position as long as it is comfortable. When you open your eyes, stretch all your limbs. This whole series of exercises, if you concentrate on them, will make you feel as though you've had a good night's rest.

*Exercises for facial muscles and scalp:*
Tense facial and scalp muscles can also cause headaches, so include these exercises to ease that tension.

1. Open and close your mouth as fast as you can (be sure your teeth aren't clenched), with your lips meeting each time. Repeat ten times.

2. Open your mouth as wide as you can, bringing your chin down as far as it will go. At the same time, open your eyes as wide as possible. Hold to the count of three. Repeat five times.

3. Place both hands on the base of the skull, putting light pressure on the scalp. Move your fingers up and down, moving the scalp as you do so. Then massage the scalp with a slow circular motion to the count of ten.

Something as simple as smiling also relaxes the facial muscles and relieves tension. A lot of tension, too, is caused by clenching the teeth. Try to be aware of this habit; unclench your teeth, open your mouth slightly, and relax.

*Shoulder relaxer:*

Tense shoulder muscles can also aggravate a tension headache. Shoulder exercises are described in the chapters on sitting and standing exercises; here is another.

1. Stand straight, feet shoulder-width apart, and shoulders back.

2. Push shoulders upward, as if you were trying to touch your ears with them.

3. Now bring your shoulders back, as if you were trying to make your shoulder blades meet, then bring the shoulders down to normal position.

4. Combine all three movements, and with a rhythmic motion, bring the shoulders up, back, and down, repeating five times.

## Going to Sleep

Sometimes when we go to bed, our minds are in a turmoil. We find we simply cannot get to sleep, and nothing seems to help as we toss and turn. Here is an exercise I have shown to many senior citizens to help them relax their minds and feel sleepy, and I use this technique myself when necessary.

1. As you lie down, let your whole body go limp. Make believe that your body is leaving the bed and floating in the air. Concentrate on that floating sensation. Whenever a random thought comes into your mind, dismiss it. Think of nothing but your body floating, until you feel a little dizzy.

2. Now open your eyes wide, then close them tightly. Repeat three times. Keep on thinking of the floating sensation.

3. Now concentrate on the pupils of your eyes. They are sinking to the back of your head. If any thought enters your mind, dismiss it. Concentrate on your pupils sinking farther and farther into the back of your head until you are aware of nothing but darkness.

4. Go back to thinking about the floating sensation again, keeping your body limp and relaxed.

5. Now move your head gently from side to side until you feel completely relaxed and sleepy.

If the exercise doesn't quite work the first time, don't give up.

Try it over again. You'll find it's an excellent way to round off a busy day and send yourself to sleep with a calm, relaxed mind and body.

One final note about sleep: If you wake in the night, and worry about getting back to sleep, try the sleep-inducing exercises I've just described. But if you can't get to sleep, don't worry. Worry creates more tension. Put your time to relaxing use—keep a book or magazine beside your bed; try knitting or embroidery.

# ELEVEN

# Special Exercises: Beauty and Weight Control

*T*oo often today the only reason people bother to exercise is because they think it's going to turn them into beauties overnight. If they are overweight, instead of cutting out calorie-loaded foods, they hope and pray that exercise alone is going to work a miracle and make them slim and trim.

Alas, it's simply not true. I will make many claims for exercise, but that is not among them. Health is the first and most important reason to exercise. I believe, however, that a person who represents the peak of well-exercised health is also beautiful. And I will claim that a regular exercise program is a wonderful aid to losing inches, whether you are a senior citizen or a young person.

What can exercise do in terms of beauty and weight control? If you look better because of exercise, if you walk straighter and glow with health, you'll find yourself getting compliments you never had before. The exercises that tone your muscles help to tighten up flabby areas of your body. Exercises for the circulation help keep your mind alert and bring a glow to your face. Exercising away stiff joints, or a stiff neck, will make you move and act years younger. All exercises, in short, benefit the way you look.

There are, however, a few specific exercises that you can do to lessen or eliminate some beauty problems caused by years of lack of exercise.

## Facial Exercises

The first thing people see when they look at us is our faces. It's from our faces that they first judge our ages, and if we haven't paid attention to what the years do to us, they'll automatically write us off as "old."

When Helen first came to my senior citizens class at an old age home, I was puzzled that such a young person was in a home for older people. She had a marvelously smooth neck and a firm chinline, and there were hardly any wrinkles on her face. From her agility and her youthful appearance, I guessed that she might be in her late fifties.

I started to show the group some facial exercises, and Helen chimed in with, "I've been doing these exercises for fifty years."

"Do you mean," asked another woman in the group, "that you've been doing exercises since you were a baby?"

Helen laughed and said, "I'm eighty-two years old."

Even though she had a fifty-year start on the rest of the group, Helen served as their model and inspiration, as far as facial exercises went.

The belief that age must show on our faces and that a double chin and hanging facial flab are inevitable results of aging is simply not true. We know that exercise can firm muscles in all parts of the body—a flabby thigh, for example—and it can do the same with flabby facial muscles.

Before you do any facial exercises, lubricate your face with a skin cream or plain petroleum jelly, to soften the tissues. Pat the face with both hands to bring blood to it and warm up the muscles for the more strenuous exercises. Facial exercises should be done every night before you go to bed and every morning when you get up (before you apply makeup, if you are a woman). Although we think of women as being more worried than men about having a beautiful and youthful face, I recommend that men do these exercises as well to help keep chinlines and facial muscles firm.

1. Stand in front of a mirror. Hold the chin in a relaxed downward position, since pushing it out and up may stretch the skin of the neck.

2. Press your lips together tightly to pull the muscles and flab on your jaws, chin, and neck up toward the upper cheeks. Hold to the count of five.

3. Now open your mouth and eyes as wide as you can, dropping the jaw down to make a long O. Hold to the count of five.

4. Alternate those two motions five times each. Your goal is to work up to at least ten times in the morning and ten at night, but start out with five times morning and night for two weeks.

5. To help erase the lines around the mouth leading to the nose, purse your lips and make movements like a fish drinking water. Repeat ten times each morning and night.

6. A marvelous way to tone facial muscles is to repeat a long Ooooooo and Ahhhhhh over and over again.

## Tightening Up Flabby Areas of the Body

We are ashamed to expose certain parts of the body because we have allowed them to get flabby. Those areas deserve our special attention. (Only those who are agile and capable of doing the exercises easily should attempt to do them.)

*Firming the abdomen:*

　　1. Sit on the floor and bring both knees in to your chest.

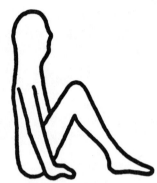

　　2. Stretch both hands out in front of you, palms down, and very slowly lean backward, lowering the body about one foot. Hold to the count of five.

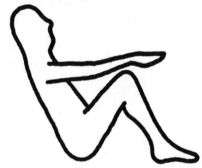

　　3. Lower the body another foot, and hold to the count of five.

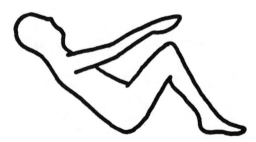

4. Keep on lowering the body a foot at a time, until you are lying on the floor. (Note that this is not an easy exercise, and should be attempted only by those who have been working steadily on a conditioning program. They, too, may have to work on this exercise for some time before perfecting it.)

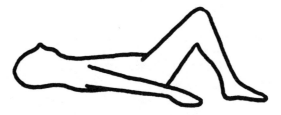

*Toning buttocks and thighs:*
When women wear pants, it is obvious whether or not they exercise. The hip and thigh present a smooth line if they have been exercised; if not, the flab will be bulging out. The outer thigh muscles, just below the hip line, can pose a special problem, even with the best-exercised individual.

1. Sit in a chair without arms. Stretch out your right leg in front of you, with your knee as straight as possible, heel on the floor.

2. Lift the leg up to the level of the seat and turn the foot all the way to the right, forcing the toes as far right as possible.

3. Contract the thigh muscles, and hold to the count of five. Repeat once. Repeat exercise with the other leg.

1. Lie on the floor on your left side, and hold your head in the palm of your left hand.

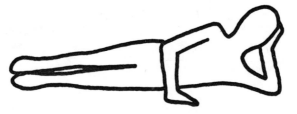

2. Lift your right leg up, keeping the knee straight, and sway it all the way to the left, into your chest.

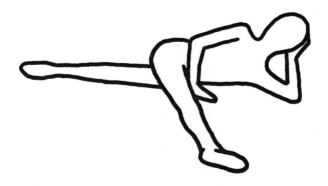

3. In slow motion, sway it all the way back behind you. Repeat five times and do the exercise with the other leg, while lying on your right side.

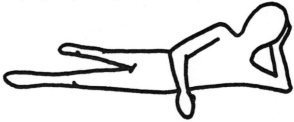

*Tightening flab on the upper back:*
When summer comes, we are often embarrassed by the flab hanging out of our bathing suits in the back. Here's an exercise to help eliminate that flab.

    1. Stand straight, feet shoulder-width apart for balance. Stretch out your right arm in front of you, with the elbow as straight as possible and the palm down.

    2. Now move the arm as far to the left as possible, so that your upper arm touches your chin; imagine you are trying to reach a distant wall on your left. Hold to the count of five and relax. Repeat five times: reach, relax, reach, relax. Repeat with the left arm reaching to the right.

*Tightening flab under the arms:*
"The day of wearing an off-the-shoulder dress or a sleeveless blouse has long passed me by," Mrs. Merton said one day in class. "My arms are so flabby I'm ashamed to show them." Here's an exercise I gave Mrs. Merton to firm up the upper arm.

    1. Stand straight, feet shoulder-width apart. Let your hands hang loosely at your sides, with the palms touching the thighs.

    2. Now imagine that someone has placed a huge weight on the back of each hand and is forcing you to lift the weight as high as you can. Raise your arms as you con-

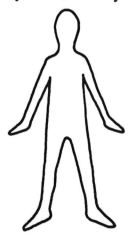

centrate on the flab you want to tighten, keeping in mind the terrific weight pressing down on your hands. As you slowly raise your arms to shoulder level, you will feel the flabby muscles in the upper arm contracting.

3. When your arms are at shoulder level, push them backward and outward as far as you can.

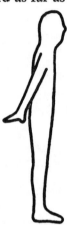

4. Release all pressure and shake your hands loosely. This is a very strenuous exercise, and should be done once, four times a day, at wide intervals.

*Trimming the waistline:*

1. Stand straight, feet shoulder-width apart, with your hands on your hips.

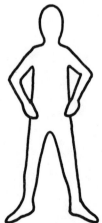

2. Turn the body and head all the way to the right, pulling your left hip upward. Feel and pull on your left side. Hold to the count of five. Now do the same exercise to the left side. Alternate sides, five times for each.

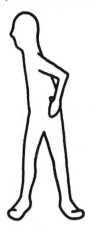

*Firming the bustline:*

Don't be duped into believing that your bust size can be increased or decreased with exercise gimmicks. Weight-lifting and certain isometric exercises can increase only *chest* size, but the cup size remains the same. For women, the only thing exercise can do is firm the bustline. In the course of overall weight loss on a reducing program, bust size can be decreased, but that has nothing to do with exercise.

1. Put both hands above your head, the right hand grasping the left elbow, and the left hand grasping the right elbow.

2. Push both elbows upward and back. Hold to the count of five. Repeat three times.

These exercises for improving the appearance of various parts of the body can be combined with your daily exercises for muscle-toning, circulation, and flexibility to help you look and feel better while you condition your body.

## Exercise and Weight Control

This is not a book on diet and nutrition, but we are bombarded with so much talk about the subject that I want to offer a few words to the senior citizen who may think that exercise alone will work miracles for overweight.

As we get older, if we are not as active as we used to be, our bodies need fewer calories. If you have not reduced your intake of food (calories) as the years have gone by, chances are that you have grown steadily heavier. With fewer calories used up in less active daily lives, the pounds pile up. A healthy, well-rounded diet is essential; chocolates, lots of bread and butter, rich desserts, and junk food snacks are not.

If you are overweight, your doctor can give you advice on dieting. You will almost always lose weight if you take in fewer calories than you use up each day.

What part does exercise play in weight control? While exercise alone will not cause significant, rapid weight loss, it does have an essential role in weight control.

Mrs. Bergstrom was on a reducing program but was discouraged because she told me, "It doesn't seem to matter how much weight I lose; I can't go below a size twelve."

I explained to her that weight loss alone wasn't going to get her into a smaller dress size automatically. Her body was flabby, and in order to tighten up that flab, she had to exercise, which would result in the loss of inches as well as pounds, and a smaller dress size.

I've seen many of my students go down two sizes without losing an ounce of weight and without changing their eating habits. What they've done is eliminate that middle-age and old-age spread that makes us bottom-heavy. They haven't done it with girdles, either; but with exercise that firms up muscles and reduces flab.

Girdles, incidentally, are a false comfort. All they do is hold together bodies that are collapsing because of flabby and weak muscles. You may think that a girdle makes you look better, but all it actually does is press the fat from below upward. It can also impair blood circulation, which none of us can afford to do.

I remember one of my friends telling me that every time she went out with her husband, she wore a complicated girdle to keep her "together."

"By the time the party was over," she said, "I could hardly wait to get to the car so I could start undressing. I'd end up walking into my house with my girdle in my hands, hoping the neighbors were fast asleep and couldn't see me in that state."

My friend went on a diet to lose weight and began an exercise program to firm up her body, "because," she told me, "I've seen women who flaunt their figures after losing a lot of weight. They look fine with their clothes on, but in a bathing suit or shorts, they look as though their bodies had been chewed up by wild animals—a lot of flab that didn't go away when the pounds did."

Many people ask me if it is true that when you exercise flab turns to muscle and that muscle weighs more than flab, so you end up gaining weight instead of losing it. Muscle does weigh more than flab, but by the time you have reached the point where, through exercise, you have gained a pound or two because of improved muscle tone, you will have lost inches in size.

Besides helping to control flab, exercise plays another part in weight control. If you have been leading a completely sedentary existence before you began to exercise, you are now using up more calories than you did before. If you don't change your eating habits, and if you keep up your exercises each day along with a brisk walk daily or several times a week, by the end of a year, you may have dropped ten or fifteen pounds. If you walk to the store instead of taking out the car each time you want groceries or a newspaper, if you walk up the stairs to your apartment instead of always taking the elevator, if you make yourself get up out of your chair and do something, you're going to be using up excess calories slowly and steadily.

On the other hand, if you insist on sitting in your chair all day, riding the elevator, driving when you could walk—if you don't, in short, exercise at all—you may be adding ten or fifteen pounds to your weight in a year's time.

What about the claim that exercise increases your appetite so that you eat more and gain weight? I firmly disagree. Most excess food consumption seems to be found in people who aren't active, and have a lot of time to think about food. Active individuals are, as a rule, too occupied to think about eating all the time. In fact, I believe that most overeaters do so out of frustration and tension. Since exercise is a miraculous tension-reliever, it helps curb your appetite instead of increasing it.

# TWELVE

# Advanced Program: Exercises for the Well-Conditioned

*N*ow that you have a basic exercise program of sitting and standing exercises, and some special exercises for specific problems, don't stop there. The exercises in this chapter are designed to give you back the youthful bounce and agility you may have lost. They will help train the muscles to react with speed. They will also help to improve the respiratory system, strengthen the heart and blood vessels, and supply the brain with oxygen necessary for it to function properly. After you have spent a few weeks or months getting your body in shape with the basic program, including muscle-toning, you should be able to gradually add these new exercises. If you are already in good condition, you should be doing both the basic exercises and these more stimulating ones right from the beginning.

Several groups of exercises are given here. Each group is sufficiently stimulating so that if you are rushed or feel like taking a day off from the other exercises, you can do that one group and obtain the maximum benefits in a short time. I don't however, recommend that you do *only* the exercises in this chapter. To make sure that all parts of the body are fully exercised, you must do all the exercises given in this book. Your exercise program ought eventually take about a half hour a day, every day. The least amount of time is a half hour three times a week—say, Monday, Wednesday, and Friday. You simply cannot exert yourself for a long period once a week and expect to get any benefit from exercise. Exercise cannot be "stored up" to last through the week.

Whenever you are about to begin exercising, and especially for these more strenuous and challenging exercises, remember your heart. The body must be warmed up slowly before you start the exercises.

I suggest that you make it a habit to begin these exercises with a slow walk around the room for about three minutes. Then walk faster for another minute, followed by a minute of walking as quickly as you can, swinging your arms as you move. Finally, taper off slowly, and walk at a more leisurely pace until your breathing is back to normal. Now stop and rock your body back and forth to loosen up the spine, then raise your arms and stretch like a cat, moving every part of your body. You are now ready to get on with the exercises.

Since the exercises are geared to stimulate blood circulation, I urge you to observe these safety precautions: Start off slowly, increase the speed of your movements until your breathing rate increases, then decrease speed until your breathing returns to normal and your body is free of fatigue.

*Never,* at the peak of exercising, decide that you deserve a rest and sit down. That could be dangerous or even fatal. Always taper off gradually. When we exercise using our legs to stimulate the blood circulation, the heart has to work harder to supply the lower extremities with the blood and energy they need to keep moving. If you stop an activity suddenly, that extra blood remains pooled in your feet and legs, and you put too great a burden on the heart, requiring it all at once to bring the blood back into normal circulation.

Imagine pumping water from an old-fashioned water pump. You start slowly, and the water comes slowly. As you speed up the pumping action, the water comes faster and faster. If you suddenly stop pumping at that point, the water that was almost to the top rushes back down into the well without coming out. However, if you keep on pumping more gently, the flow of water gradually decreases until you stop.

The same principle applies to the heart. During exercise, the heart is pumping blood to the moving legs. In order to help the heart bring up the blood from the lower extremities safely, you taper off your activities with a continuous motion of the entire body, including gentle pumping motions with both arms.

## *Group One*

Since this exercise requires balancing as well as speed, it may feel a little awkward at first, as well as tiring. If that is the case, work up to it slowly.

1. Stand with shoulders bent forward.

2. With as much speed as you can manage, bring your left knee up and into your chest and down, grabbing the knee with both hands as it comes up and letting go of it as it goes down.

3. Now do the same with the right knee, and continue alternating knees, up and down, as quickly as you can, as many times as you can, until your breathing rate increases markedly, but never to the point where you have to gasp for breath.

4. Slow down your body by walking about the room slowly, raising one hand over your head and down and then the other. (Again, the hands act as a pump to aid the heart.) Keep walking until your body is completely relaxed and your breathing is back to normal.

### Group Two

1. Stand with shoulders limp and relaxed. Bend down, and keeping the body bent over at the waist, bounce the body downwards, touching the toes, ten times.

2. Stand up straight, with your hands on your hips, lean to the right and bounce the body ten times. Now lean to the left and repeat.

3. Tilt the body and shoulders backward (but don't tilt head), and bounce backward to the count of ten.

4. Repeat the toe touch, this time to the count of nine, and the bouncing motion to the right, left, and back, also to the count of nine.

5. Repeat the whole routine, to the count of eight, then seven, and so forth, until you reach one. If you feel genuinely exhausted before you get to one (it will take time to build up to the complete exercise), don't stop suddenly.

6. Whenever you decide you have done enough of this exercise, walk about slowly, hands pumping in the air, until your breathing returns to normal.

### Group Three

1. Start off with a slow walk around the room for five minutes, increasing your speed until you are moving as fast as you can. Swing your arms as you walk. Keep this up for as much as seven minutes. (When you walk, remember to take a long stride, throwing your legs out from your hips, not the knees. Let your hips propel the motion.)

2. Skip around a table or around the room until you are breathing heavily, but not so much that you have to gasp for breath.

3. Now walk briskly, decreasing your speed. Walk until your body feels relaxed and your breathing is back to normal.

4. Increase your walking again to capacity speed for a few minutes.

5. Hop forward on both feet at once, five times.

6. Walk a minute or two at a fast rate.

7. Hop again to the count of five.

8. Walk at a fast rate, moving your hands.

9. Start slowing down your walk gradually, until your body has completely cooled off and you are breathing normally.

## *Morning Routine*

Some of us prefer to exercise for a few minutes early in the morning. Starting off the day with a refreshed and stimulated mind and body can be a great help to you in getting through your daily routine. It's a way to get charged up and relaxed at the same time.

Here is a morning exercise routine for those in good physical condition. It may also be used by those who are working on conditioning their bodies with the other exercises in this book. But those individuals should start off slowly, with fewer repetitions of each activity, until they catch up. Remember how to get out of bed so as not to shock your system by sudden activity.

1. In my years of teaching exercise, I have found that the knees are the part of the body most vulnerable to injury. Every exercise program I give includes an exercise to strengthen kneecaps. Stand straight and contract the kneecaps. Hold to the count of five. Do this ten times. Always do exercises that require contraction of muscles when the blood circulation is not too stimulated by activity. In other

words, do this exercise at the beginning of your morning routine before you do anything else.

2. Walk around the room, counting as you walk, between three hundred and five hundred steps.

3. Stand straight and touch your toes, straighten up, touch toes. Repeat twenty times. If you have back problems, consult your doctor. It is advisable when touching your toes to bend the knees to relieve pressure on the spine.

4. Raise your hands above your head and stretch each hand alternately toward the ceiling, as though you were pushing upward from the hips, trying to grow a little. Repeat ten times for each hand.

5. Put both hands on the top of the head, elbows close to the head, and bend the whole body to the right from the waist. Hold to the count of five. Stand upright, and bend to the left. Repeat the series of motions ten times.

6. Stand straight with legs apart. Bend your knees in a forward position, lowering the body, and return to standing position. Repeat five times.

7. Stand straight. Kick the right leg out to the side and bring it back to position. Repeat with the left leg. With a fast, rhythmic motion, alternate right and left legs, ten times for each.

8. Stand with your arms stretched out in front of you, palms down. Kick up the left leg in front of you so that your toes touch the left hand. Repeat with the right leg. Alternate right and left legs, with a brisk, rhythmic motion, ten times for each leg. Now repeat the exercise, only this time have the left toes touch the right hand, the right toes the left, ten times for each. (This exercise requires good coordination and balance, so you may have to practice it for a while until you are able to do it the suggested number of times.)

9. If you have done all of these exercises, your pulse rate will probably have risen, so don't stop suddenly. Walk

around the room gently, keeping your arms in motion, until your breathing is back to normal.

## *Music for Exercise*

If you want to enjoy yourself more when you exercise, do it to music. "There's nothing so stirring as music that reaches the soul," eighty-five-year-old Louise is always telling people. "I put on my favorite record for twenty minutes each day and lose myself in the music while I exercise."

Music reaches everyone. It stirs emotions in people who have been given up as hopeless, it brings to their feet those who would otherwise refuse to exercise.

About two years ago, I used to see Mr. Cohen every week in an old age home where I conducted a fitness class. He never showed any interest in our activities. Instead, he had a spot near a window where he sat and stared endlessly out into space. Even a "good morning" produced only a blank stare from him.

On day in my class, where I often used all kinds of ethnic music as background for exercises, I put on a recording of Chassidic music that accompanies a traditional Jewish dance. And a miracle happened. Mr. Cohen, with smiling eyes, edged toward the center of the exercise group, and with great expression and emotion, performed a Chassidic dance. It took only music to stir up Mr. Cohen's memories and get him out of his chair.

In another home, Mr. McCormack, who was always uninterested in everything that went on around him, got up suddenly at one of the exercise sessions with music, performed a tap dance for the amazed and delighted group, and did a very professional job of it.

Try using music at home when you exercise. Put on a march, or a nostalgic tune. You might turn on the radio and take a chance on whatever is playing, adapting your movements to fit the music. You don't even have to do a formal exercise. Just move every part of the body, as if you wanted to separate it into different sections, and work on different parts, so that no one part will get too tired. Moving to music will often relieve your pent-up tensions, too, and of course it stimulates the blood circulation. Since music plays a big part in group exercise activities, you may want to turn to the chapters on groups for other suggestions for using music when you exercise.

## *Other Physical Activities*

If you've been exercising for a while and want to get involved in activities that exercise your body but are more than simple at-home, in-place exercises, there are plenty of ways to do so. A physically fit senior citizen can participate in such sports as swimming or bicycling. Swimming, for example, is an excellent exercise, and one of the safest. The movements are rhythmic and steady, and stimulate every part of the body. If there is a pool in your community, perhaps at the local Y, by all means go swimming. For total fitness, a now-and-then swimmer might want to make it a regular part of the exercise program, perhaps three times a week (and always with a lifeguard present).

A word of caution, however. In our modern society, we hear a lot about sports like tennis and jogging that suddenly become fashionable. Nobody denies the need for regular exercise at any age. Middle-aged persons, young men and women, teenagers, all are urged to maintain their physical fitness. But a lot of harm can come to weekend athletes and enthusiasts who do not heed safety precautions before embarking on exercise programs. This is especially true for senior citizens. Just because you have started out on a conditioning program, it does not mean that you are fit to rush out onto a tennis court and engage in an hour of fast tennis with a youthful instructor who plays every day of the year.

If you want to get involved in a sport, start slowly and with your doctor's approval. Don't give up regular daily exercise and try to replace it with vigorous but sporadic athletics. Condition the body first with the exercises I have given, and *then* look into a sport.

And use common sense. Don't try to compete beyond your abilities. I never urge senior citizens as a group to undertake strenuous sports activities. They are really suitable only for those who are completely fit to undertake them.

## Jogging

I have a lot of reservations about jogging programs for senior citizens. It is true that jogging, if all the safety precautions are adhered to, is one of the best exercises for strengthening the heart, lungs, and blood vessels. It is also a tremendous stamina-builder.

However, most joggers are not sufficiently educated in the ways to jog safely. If it is done safely, it has many assets; if it is done improperly, it can be a killer. Sporadic jogging may put fatal strain on the heart instead of making it stronger. I believe firmly in moderation in any exercise you undertake. Jogging is extremely strenuous, so I strongly recommend that you do not include it in your choice of exercises.

If you are already a regular jogger and you and your doctor feel that it is good for you, by all means continue. However, I have seen joggers become so enthusiastic once they start that they pay no attention to moderation. For instance, if your heart beats about eighty times per minute at rest, by constant jogging, you might reduce your heartbeat to, say, sixty-five beats per minute. That is a moderate goal, and in my opinion, you shouldn't force your body to jog harder in order to bring your pulse rate lower still.

Also, what many joggers and exercise enthusiasts don't

realize, until it is too late, is that in jogging hard to strengthen the heart, they are wearing out their joints, especially the hip and knee joints, which are vulnerable to injury, something we cannot afford in later years. Jogging in place is the greatest culprit, since it can affect the knee joint. I have many friends who found out the hard way. Because they wanted a stronger heart, they pushed themselves so much they ended up with damaged knees. Now they are no longer able to jog, and their hearts suffer, as well as their knee joints. The constant pounding involved in jogging may also injure internal organs.

For the senior citizen, then, I strongly recommend a walking program instead of jogging. You can increase your capacity and speed, and this gives the heart plenty of exercise. If you insist on jogging, incorporate five minutes of jogging in the course of a brisk half-hour walk. Start out walking, jog a few steps, and return to walking. At first, do no more than a few jogging steps, and only gradually increase your time to about five minutes out of your half hour. Give yourself several months to reach this amount of time, particularly if you are totally unaccustomed to jogging.

When you do jog, don't overexert yourself. Wear light clothing and good shoes designed for the activity, and never jog in very hot or very cold weather. Don't do your jogging on concrete sidewalks or in the road. Use a jogging track that is designed especially for running, or a dirt or grass surface.

## Yoga

I have a yoga teacher who is in her sixties. Her body is more flexible than students who are half her age, and I have no doubt that she will be doing yoga exercises a decade from now. She is a remarkable example of the benefits of yoga. Yet it is another activity that I cannot recommend whole-heartedly for senior citizens.

If you are already doing yoga and find it beneficial and relaxing, there is no reason why you shouldn't continue. Doing any exercise safely is better than doing no exercise at all. However, I do not consider yoga a complete exercise. Although it is a marvelous muscle-toner, it does very little to strengthen the heart or the respiratory system. Nor does it prepare the body to fight everyday fatigue. It is not the stamina- or agility-builder I want all readers of this book to have. I have encountered many people in my regular classes for both younger and older persons who have been participating in yoga programs. It seems that a walk for a period of five minutes brings their heart rate up to an alarming 140 beats per minute, which indicates to me that yoga does not do an efficient conditioning job on the whole body.

If you have decided to join a yoga class anyhow, make sure that the yoga teacher is experienced and has enough sensitivity to understand the initial limitations of a senior citizen just starting out. Yoga is a strenuous muscle-toner, and if overdone, may lay you up for weeks. Be sure, also, that you reread the chapter on breathing earlier in this book. I have seen many yoga students get dizzy and faint from hyperventilation after a yoga breathing session. I advise you strongly not to tamper with your regular breathing habits. I would also suggest that you eliminate headstands.

My advice to yoga participants is: Go on with it, but if you want to benefit the whole body and the mind and to stimulate the blood circulation, make it a habit to take a brisk walk each day in addition to yoga exercises.

## Isometrics

Any exercise can have dangers if you don't know how to do it properly. However, it is especially important to warn against the dangers of isometric exercises. If you contract a muscle or a group of muscles, if you make a tight fist and press one muscle against another, or if you press muscles against an object when neither muscles nor object moves, that is an isometric. Isometric exercises have a place in certain exercise programs, and some of the exercises included in this book are isometric, particularly in the Miracle Box exercises.

Senior citizens and the middle-aged must perform them with care, following instructions exactly, not exceeding the count given for each. The need for special care lies in the fact that when a muscle is contracted, the blood flow through that muscle is reduced or cut off, which is not always good for older people. You would be wise to get your doctor's advice before doing any isometric exercises.

## THIRTEEN

# The Miracle Box

*M*ONOTONY is the worst part of exercising. We start off enthusiastically for a week or two, but as time goes by, we find our interest beginning to dull. It gets harder and harder to do the prescribed exercises.

The one thing senior citizens must never do is allow themselves to sink back into a sedentary existence. Exercise must become part of their way of life. Those excuses for not exercising —"I'm too tired today." "I exercised a lot yesterday." "Nothing helps me any more, I'm too old."—have no validity. You're never too old; yesterday's exercises aren't going to help you today, or tomorrow, or in the years to come.

Even if you have the exercise habit, there are going to be times when you are bored. What do you do about it? Some strong-willed people who have been thoroughly educated to the benefits of exercise don't need any help to keep exercising regularly. But most of us need a little help from time to time, something that might add a little interest to the process. For that reason, I have put together a Miracle Box.

The Miracle Box holds exercise miracles—and a handful of simple objects found in every household or readily obtained for very little expense. With the Miracle Box, you'll be able to vary your exercises so that you will never get bored. You may wish to use only one or two of the objects listed, or you can get together everything mentioned. Since the exercises using the contents of the Miracle Box are designed to be done while sitting in a chair, you can do them while watching television, or at intervals while reading, knitting, or relaxing.

Since some of the exercises in the Miracle Box are isometric (requiring contraction of a number of muscles and resistance), I ask you to read carefully the specific instructions for each one of the moves. Isometric exercises are strenuous, and you must take special precautions with them. Do not exceed the prescribed count for holding each exercise, and do not exceed the number of times each exercise is to be performed. Don't alter your regular breathing while you are holding to a given count, and above all, don't hold your breath.

## *Items for Miracle Box*

Get a small box or carton—even an unused wastepaper basket will do—and collect the following items:

1. A soft rubber ball, two inches in diameter
2. A ball, eight to ten inches in diameter (beach ball, light rubber ball)
3. A piece of two-inch-wide elastic, about a yard long, sewed together at the ends to form a loop
4. Two medium-sized hardcover books
5. A small pail with a handle (such as a child uses at the beach) or a pocketbook with handles
6. A bucket
7. Two sixteen-ounce cans of food

8. Lupolastic—a two-inch wide piece of elastic, three and a half feet long, with loops large enough for your hands sewn at each end.

Keep the Miracle Box in a corner of your living room, so that you can take out items whenever you are not otherwise occupied, and do a few exercises.

## Exercises with Miracle Box

*Small rubber ball:*
1. Hold the ball in the palm of your hand.
2. Squeeze it to the count of three and release. Repeat four times with each hand.

That strengthens the muscles in the fingers, hands, and wrists. Do this exercise frequently, particularly if you have a problem with weak hands.

*Eight-inch ball:*
This exercise strengthens the back of the hand, the wrist, and the arm.
1. Hold the ball in front of you between the palms of your hands, keeping your hands flat on the ball.
2. Press the ball with both hands as hard as you can, putting most of the pressure on the heel of your hands. Squeeze to the count of five. Repeat four times.

*Eight-inch ball, finger exercises:*
This is an exercise to strengthen fingers, the joints in the hands, the wrists and the arms.
1. Grip the ball with the fingers of both hands. Have your fingers curved around the ball, not flat against it.
2. With fingers on the ball and hands arched, press the fingers into the ball and hold to the count of three. Repeat four times, relaxing between each.

*Lupolastic:*

> 1. Sit in a chair. (If you are steady enough, you can stand.) Put the elastic under your feet, and hold the loops with your hands.

> 2. Relax shoulders, and pull on the elastic, first with one hand, then the other, up and to the side.

*Ball-and-pail exercise for coordination:*

This simple exercise is excellent for improving coordination. There are several ways to do it, depending on your physical condition. You must decide how able you are when you start out. Here is the basic exercise:

> 1. Place bucket about five feet away from your chair, and sit in the chair with the eight-inch ball.

> 2. Toss the ball into the bucket. If you consistently hit the bull's-eye, move the bucket farther away. If you still find this too easy, try it with the small pail and the small rubber ball, starting out with the pail close to the chair, moving it away as you start getting more accurate. If you find it difficult to get the ball in the pail on your first few tries, don't get discouraged. Keep trying until you are proficient.

You may also do this exercise standing up, if you are able. That way is marvelous exercise for the whole body, as you are standing, walking, and bending to retrieve the ball.

If you feel that a lack of balance or agility will hinder you in bending down and picking up missed balls, roll the ball back to the chair with your feet, sit, and pick the ball up from a sitting position. You can also use a dustpan with a long handle and a broom for retrieving the ball.

The advantage of this exercise, besides helping coordination, is that it requires you to move about and gives you an opportunity to practice getting up from a chair.

*Ball exercise with friend, spouse, grandchild:*

Tossing the eight-inch ball back and forth to a friend, your spouse, or a grandchild is an excellent way to help coordination. It's fun as well, and may give you a welcome opportunity to enjoy some time with grandchildren.

*Elastic ring:*
This exercise, repeated frequently, will strengthen the whole hand.

    1. Put both hands inside the loop of elastic.

    2. Stretch the loop with the backs of your hands. Hold to the count of three, and relax the elastic. Repeat four times.

*Two books, for strength:*
If your hands and arms are weak, start off using two small hardcover books. If you are able, however, you should start with medium-sized ones, then graduate to heavier books as your strength increases. This exercise promotes strength and flexibility in the arms, shoulders, and upper back.

    1. Hold a book in each hand, and raise both arms above your head, as if you wanted to reach the ceiling.

    2. Lower the right hand and try to touch the right shoulder with the book. Do the same with your left hand.

    3. Raise both hands again, still holding the books, and repeat the whole procedure five times, using a rhythmic motion.

*Two cans of food, for strength:*
This exercise uses two sixteen-ounce cans of food to strengthen shoulders, lower and upper back, and abdominal muscles. As your strength increases, you can substitute heavier cans, the twenty-eight-ounce or thirty-two-ounce size. If you do not feel physically able to start out with sixteen-ounce cans, you can use smaller cans and graduate to larger sizes as you get stronger.

    1. Sit in a chair, with your feet twelve inches apart.

    2. Place the cans on the floor in front of you, about the distance your arms can reach.

3. With the body bent forward, grasp the can on the right with the right hand and raise it to shoulder level. Set it down and repeat five times. Now do the same with the left can and hand.

*Small pail or pocketbook, and can of food, for feet:*
For this exercise, use a small pail with a handle or a pocketbook with handles. Place a can of food in the pail or pocketbook. You can start out with a small can and go up to a sixteen-ounce can or larger as you feel your feet getting stronger.

1. Sit straight in a chair, with your hips and shoulders touching the back.

2. Place the pail in front of you on the floor, as far from you as the distance your leg reaches when stretched out.

3. Now stretch out your right leg and slip your foot under the handle or loop so that it rests in the middle of your foot.

4. With toes pointing straight ahead and your knee as straight as possible, slowly lift the pail off the floor with your foot, as high as you can. Hold to the count of four. Repeat once. Repeat the exercise with your other foot.

This exercise will strengthen the muscles in your feet, ankles, legs, knees, thighs, and abdomen.

## Other Exercise Devices

The objects found in the Miracle Box will help take the monotony out of exercising at home. They have the great advantage of being inexpensive and easy to obtain, as commercial devices frequently are not, and they and the exercises given in this book are all you need for a complete fitness program.

As I said earlier, I don't recommend that senior citizens purchase the expensive exercise devices we often see advertised on television and in magazines. They are not always suitable for older persons who are not in good physical condition. Some of them require you to lie on the floor and pull and stretch muscles that haven't been used for years.

I do recommend, however, a stationary indoor bicycle, if you can afford one. A stationary bicycle is a safe device for persons of all ages, provided it is low with a firm platform so that it does not tip and so that senior citizens don't have to climb up onto it. The pedaling motion is excellent exercise, particularly if you continue the other toning, circulatory, and flexibility exercises I have given.

My friend Mark, who is nearly seventy, is now semi retired, but he keeps a little office where he goes for part of the day to do a little business and to play cards with his cronies who drop in. It's amusing to see Mark concentrating on his cards as he pedals away furiously on his stationary bicycle. He's in much better shape than his card-playing friends who do nothing but sit.

Even if you are a regular bicycle-rider and ride outdoors whenever you can, there will be days when the weather is bad and you aren't able to get out. Your stationary indoor bicycle doesn't depend on the weather, and you can exercise on it any time you want.

My only warning is that you start out slowly if you are unaccustomed to bike-riding, testing your body to see how much of that kind of exercise you can take at one time. Be sure to ease off slowly, following the same principles of tapering off that you would in doing any vigorous exercise.

Do a few minutes of bicycling the first time, and wait until the next day to see if you are stiff and sore. If you are not, increase your time daily until your body tells you that you have reached your limit. After that limit is reached, do about the same amount of pedaling for the next few days; then challenge yourself to increase your time by a minute or two. Keep on increasing your time as you grow stronger, extending your limit gradually to get the full benefit of this exercise.

# FOURTEEN

# Starting a Group Exercise Program

**D**AILY exercising does take a lot of will power. But daily exercise is a must, especially for senior citizens, to maintain vigor, health, a sense of well-being, and independence.

You must exercise on a regular basis: daily if possible, three times a week at the very least, but never just two hours now and then on the weekend. Such a practice not only doesn't work, it's dangerous.

Most of us need an incentive to continue an exercise program faithfully over months and years. There is always an excuse if we want to think of a way to get out of exercising. You may be able to think up lots of good excuses, but I can answer with an equal number of good reasons why exercise is essential. If, for example, you have lost the use of one limb, there is all the more reason to exercise to preserve the strength and mobility of the remaining limb. Perhaps you have a touch of arthritis, and your doctor has told you to exercise the affected joints. It is convenient to argue with yourself that if you move your joints they will hurt, and there's no point in hurting yourself. Yet many doctors have said that if you do *not* move those joints, the chances are that they will become progressively more crippled.

What incentive, then, will help you keep exercising, once you've passed the initial stages and it gets repetitious? I strongly suggest that you try forming a group, made up of a couple of your next-door neighbors in your age group, or some of the senior citizens in your community. A once-a-week meeting in your home, your apartment, the recreational room provided at a community center, or your church or temple, will add another dimension to your efforts to stay healthy through exercise. An exercise group not only gives you the incentive you need to keep on exercising at home, it also helps remove any boredom. You also will be sharing a common goal with your friends: keeping alert and healthy. And, of course, the group can quickly turn into an enjoyable social occasion.

A large part of my experience has been in dealing with group exercise. The suggestions and principles I have to offer have been tested over and over again with thousands of senior citizens. If you are a senior citizen interested in getting friends together for an exercise group, or if you are a younger person in charge of running such a group for older persons, I hope you will heed my comments, and benefit from my experience.

## *Starting a Group*

Loneliness is a shadow that can fall not only on the aged but also on all of us. It breeds unhappiness, it makes us feel useless and unwanted, and most unbearable of all, it gives us fear. I fear facing an empty day, without plans or people, with nothing to look forward to. Too many older persons face empty days, that kind of loneliness, every day of their lives.

Nina, who had recently joined an exercise class of mine, told me, "My greatest enemy is time. It mocks me day and night, reminding me how useless I have become."

I compare her with another class member, Grace, who had many of the same problems as Nina, but had stopped brooding about them by keeping busy and involved, looking forward to each day with zest and eagerness. "I take pride in doing my good deeds each day," Grace used to say, "and in being the belle of the ball at every function."

Getting the two women together at our weekly classes showed Nina how to fight her loneliness, and how to get involved and more interested in life.

An exercise group that you and three or four friends start together can make the difference between staying at home alone and spending time profitably. Perhaps you could plan to exercise at a different home two or three times a week. The meetings could be combined with refreshments or lunch after you have done your exercises.

In the earlier chapters of this book, I have given you an exercise program that starts with preventive activities like sitting and standing safely. Everyone in the group should be completely familiar with these activities.

Before you and your group start to exercise, everyone should be sure to get the doctor's O.K. to participate. The group cannot take responsibility for the individuals in it. You are all adults and you must be responsible for yourself and your safety. Perhaps there will be certain medical restrictions on one or another individual's activities, but most doctors will encourage their patients to participate in exercise programs.

It is important that you start off your group program slowly. A person who has read through this book understands how to allow the body to be the judge of one's limits. Each motion must at first be executed with great caution, letting the body feel the movement, and letting it decide whether the motion can be completed without discomfort.

In any group, some people will be better able to exercise than others. The point of exercising is not to compete with your neighbor but to help your own body. Lift the leg an inch off the floor today; tomorrow you may be able to lift it two inches.

Don't be too anxious to help the other participants in the group. If you can lift your leg all the way up, and your neighbor can't, that means your joints and muscles are in better condition. You will be doing your friend no favors if you try to force brittle bones and inflexible joints to do something they aren't capable of. Let everyone exercise at his or her own rate and level. If you feel exhausted or out of breath, stop for a while, and pick up with the next exercise. Don't worry that others may be doing all the exercises with ease. It takes time to get your body into shape, and you'll catch up if you don't press yourself dangerously.

Choose a leader for each session. It might be more rewarding to have a different person conduct the group each time. Each person would then have a chance to go over the exercises and prepare in advance a program for the session he or she is going to lead.

If you have a large group interested in getting together for exercise, try to find a room suitable for your activities at a local senior citizens center, church, temple, or school. (When other older people hear about your group, they'll be eager to join.) Some senior citizens centers have an activities director who might take charge of forming an exercise group, but don't let the lack of an official person "in charge" keep you from getting a group going. You can do it yourself, and it's in your best interest to do so.

Part of the fun of getting a group together is the opportunity to laugh and enjoy the company of others with similar interests. You have the chance to express yourself, and it doesn't matter what kinds of talents you have—they will be put to good use. A group may bring together people of different ethnic backgrounds, for example, and offer a chance to share others' heritage of music and dance.

### *Being a Group Leader*

To be a group leader, you have to follow a few rules, but there is nothing difficult about it even if you are inexperienced. Read and understand the exercises and warnings about exercise I've already given. You should, ideally, be engaged in an at-home exercise program, such as those I've outlined earlier. You must understand that everyone should be allowed to proceed at his or her own pace; the important thing is that everyone participate. You must encourage all participants to observe the necessary safety precautions; to listen to their bodies; not to overexert; to use common sense in sitting, standing, and exercising.

You must allow everyone in the group to contribute ideas. If someone has a funny story or a joke, let him or her tell it—it's part of the fun of having a group—but you must never forget that your common goal is to achieve physical fitness. Conversation creates a good atmosphere, but you aren't there to be an audience for a good talker or an amateur comedian. You have to be able to get back to exercising, and that sometimes requires diplomacy on the part of the leader. Perhaps you'll have to say to an overtalkative group member, "Let's do one more exercise, and while we relax afterward, you tell us your story."

But don't forget that laughter is important. Senior citizens have a vast store of tales to tell, some of them having to do with exercise. Mrs. Banion, for example, told one of my groups a story that had us laughing throughout the session: "Mr. Jones is a wonderful young man. He is the recreational director at a senior citizens hotel where I lived for a while. He was about as old as my grandson. At a fitness class, he told the fifty of us sitting there to do this exercise every morning: stand in front of the mirror and wiggle and writhe and look at ourselves and say, 'You are so beautiful, you are so lovely, you are so beautiful.' We all thought this was pretty funny, and then someone spoke up from the back of the room. 'Mr. Jones,' she said, 'when should we tell the mirror how beautiful we are—before or after we put our teeth in?' "

A good group leader will enjoy stories like this one as much as the rest of the group.

If several people in the group are taking turns being the leader, you'll get further each time if the leader has prepared the program in advance. The hour you've set aside to exercise as a group won't be wasted in trying to decide what to do. (See the next chapter for suggestions on developing a group program.)

The important thing is that everyone understands the purpose of getting a group together in the first place. You all have an interest in exercising; you all know that exercise, whether alone or in a group, will help you achieve greater physical fitness and independence in your later years. You understand that daily exercise at home is a must, as are brisk walks each day, while a weekly or twice-weekly exercise group adds interest to the program you've mapped out for yourself.

Your group, whether it consists of two or three neighbors or fifty older residents of your town or city, is sharing an important experience. You are making yourself stronger and healthier, and you are setting a fine example for younger people. Your children and grandchildren have the example of senior citizens getting together and working at doing something to help themselves.

# FIFTEEN

# A Group Exercise Program

*T*HE do's and don'ts of group exercises are the same as for individual exercises: wear light clothing that doesn't restrict circulation (no tight girdles, tight shoes, or heavy clothing that doesn't allow body heat to escape). Be sure the room is cool and well ventilated. Place chairs on a nonslippery surface, and in a group, be sure they are far enough apart so that everyone has room to stretch out arms and legs without poking someone's eye out or causing someone to trip. Make sure that shopping bags and pocketbooks are out of the way.

The participants should put their chairs in a circle with the leader in front so that everyone has a good view of him or her. At the same time the leader has personal contact with every participant. Particularly in the early stages of a group fitness program, it is important to start out talking a little about the benefits of exercise. Some of the group may not be as well educated about the value of exercise as others, and everyone should be made equally concerned about what you are going to be doing. It also helps the group concentrate on the purpose of getting together. Everyone should be encouraged to read the earlier chapters of this book and to work on the program of individual at-home exercise.

The leader should be sure that everyone knows how to sit properly, stand up correctly, and so forth. The early sessions might consist of helping each other learn how to sit and stand, checking each other's posture, and perhaps describing personal exercise programs.

Other than being certain that everyone is physically capable to join in (having the doctor's approval), no one should get involved in medical questions. You can talk about your aches and pains if you like (although I don't suggest it), but it's wrong to try to answer your friends' medical questions. Leave that to a physician.

## The Pattern for Group Exercise

You should follow an overall pattern of exercise in a group where people often have differing levels of ability and agility. There is no point in having one person who is fitter than the others dominate the group, and perhaps tire them out or even discourage them. There is no sense of accomplishment if the least fit member holds everyone in the group back. Everyone should feel free to exercise at his or her own level, while still remaining part of the group and sharing in all the activities.

The pattern is to alternate stimulating exercises with relaxing ones. For example, the first exercises should be relaxing ones that warm up the body, followed by exercises that put all the joints through slow-motion activity, then some relaxing exercises, then more stimulating exercises, ending with tapering-off activity, or perhaps a not-too-tiring dance or march.

Within the pattern, you should try to use every part of the body, so that you will get the most out of your session togehter. In planning the day's program, you can follow the suggestions given in this chapter, where I have outlined a program you can use. Or you can vary this program with other exercises found throughout the book, including perhaps some found in the Miracle Box.

## *Exercises for a Group Program*

A successful group leader never loses contact with the individual members of the group. This has been, I think, the key to my success. The group leader is, in effect, the host or hostess, as well as leader of the exercises, and you will have a more effective group if you keep the double role in mind.

*Coordination:*
The leader may start off by throwing an eight- or ten-inch lightweight ball back and forth to each participant seated or standing in a semicircle. That will help coordination and the hands and fingers. Most of all, it gives the leader a chance to greet and smile personally at each person in the group.

*Warmup—gentle exercises:*
Now you can warm up the body with very gentle exercises using, if possible, slow-tempo music such as "They Call the Wind Maria." It's fun, too, to use some nostalgic music from the past which the group can identify with.

1. Sit in the chair, both legs resting firmly on the floor, relax the shoulders, bending them slightly forward.
2. Stretch the right leg out in front with the heel resting on the floor.
3. To the tempo of the music, move the whole leg from right to left, with the heel touching the floor the whole time, to the count of five. Repeat with other leg.

1. Sit straight in the chair and stretch out right arm to the side at shoulder level.

2. To the tempo of the music, touch left shoulder with right hand and back to original position. Repeat five times. Repeat with left hand.

1. Sit straight in chair, shoulders straight.

2. To the tempo of the music, lift the right shoulder up toward the right ear as far as possible and bring it down.

3. Repeat with left shoulder. Alternating shoulders, repeat five times for each.

1. Sit in chair, feet on floor, knees about a foot apart. Bend both elbows and touch right fingertips to right shoulder, left fingertips to left.

2. Keeping this position, bend forward (don't bring the head down below heart level, to prevent dizziness), and with shoulders bent, to the tempo of the music try to touch right elbow to right knee, left elbow to left knee.

3. Alternate elbows, touching each knee five times.

1. Sit in chair, both feet touching the floor, shoulders relaxed and slightly bent forward.

2. Stretch out right leg in front as far as possible, heel resting on floor.

3. To the tempo of the music, lift the leg up, bend the knee, and bring the foot all the way back under the chair, landing on the toe.

4. Repeat five times with right leg, then five times with left leg.

1. Sit in chair, shoulders slightly bent forward.

2. Stretch out both hands, palms down, keeping elbows as straight as possible and fingers pointing straight ahead.

3. To the tempo of the music, turn palms up, then down, repeating the exercise five times.

1. Sit in chair, feet on floor, knees bent, and shoulders bent forward.

2. To the tempo of the music, bring the knees apart as far as possible, then together again. Repeat five times.

1. Sit in chair, both feet firmly on the floor, shoulders bent forward.

2. Stretch both hands out, palms up.

3. To the tempo of the music, touch shoulders with fingertips, bringing hands in and out. Rock the body back and forth with the movement of the hands and arms. Repeat five times.

If the music is still playing when the group completes the eight positions, the leader can go back and choose one or two of the positions to repeat again until the music ends.

*Joints:*

Now the leader should have the group do a series of exercises for the joints. Since these exercises need a lot of concentration, leave out the music.

*To loosen up kneecaps, thighs, buttocks:*

1. Sit straight in chair, shoulders relaxed. Bring left knee up and all the way into the chest, using the hands if necessary.

2. Stretch the leg all the way out in slow motion, with knee as straight as possible, then lower leg to floor in slow motion. Repeat five times. Repeat with right leg.

*To loosen up spine and midsection:*

1. Pretend that the chair is a rocking chair.

2. Rock the body forward and backward very gently. Repeat ten times.

*For hands, fingers, wrists, and elbows:*

Do as many of the hand and finger exercises in Chapter Eight as you have time for. The group should learn how to do all of them, because hand exercises are among the easiest to do at home at odd hours of the day.

*Sitting exercises to stimulate circulation:*

Put a short, fairly fast piece of music on the record player. The order of activities may be varied according to the wishes of the leader, and it's a good idea to add your own movements. Everyone in the group might suggest a movement and adapt it to the music, keeping in mind that every joint should get its fair share of motion. Some finger-snapping and hand-clapping is included to break up the constant movement of the body.

1. Thrust one hand out, then the other, as if boxing, using the whole body.

2. Lift up right knee, put leg down, then lift left knee.

3. Snap fingers for a moment or two.

4. Combine lifting knees and raising hands simultaneously (left knee, left hand, etc.).

5. Tilt shoulders back a little and tap feet in time to music, first right foot, then left.

6. Kick left heel out in front, heel touching floor, bring foot back on toe. Alternate right and left feet.

7. Feet close to the chair, knees and feet a few inches apart. Bounce toes together and apart.

8. Stretch out both hands, palms down, and open and close fingers.

9. Kick out right foot, heel touching floor, and at the same time stretch out right hand. Back to position, and repeat with left foot and hand. Alternate right and left a few times.

10. End with clapping.

*Music for pleasure and relaxation:*
Now the group may be ready to relax to some soft music, perhaps swaying the body gently in time to it, either sitting or standing and moving about slowly. You might even sing if you like.
Everyone should be encouraged to move, and to put a smile on,
which not only is pleasant, but also relaxes the facial muscles
and relieves tension.

*Standing exercises:*
Remember that for standing exercises, each person should
stand behind a chair in case anyone loses his or her balance.
Don't stand on a slippery surface; stand on a carpet or skid-
proof rug if possible. Make sure there are no obstacles like
pocketbooks for people to trip over. No one should be wearing
high heels, which throws balance off. Group members should
wear flat shoes or take their shoes off. For additional safety and
balance, always stand with feet shoulder-width apart.

It is the leader's responsibility to remind the group at the end
of the standing exercises to turn around and make sure the
chairs are there before sitting down (chairs get moved out of
place during exercise).

*To loosen up kneecaps:*
    1. Stand straight, feet about a foot apart, hands stretched
out for balance.
    2. Bend knees and straighten up with a bouncing
motion. Repeat five times.

*To stretch:*
    1. Stand straight, feet shoulder-width apart. Raise both
hands above the head.
    2. With the right hand, reach for the ceiling and feel the
stretch on the right side. Relax hand, keeping it raised
above head, and repeat stretching motion with left hand.
Repeat five times with each hand.

3. Now stretch both hands toward ceiling, hold to the count of three, and relax.

*For shoulders and elbows:*

1. Stand straight, feet shoulder-width apart, with arms stretched out to the side at shoulder level, palms up.

2. With a rhythmic motion, bend the right elbow and touch the top of the head with the right hand. Swing the right hand back to position, and repeat with left hand. Alternate right and left hands, five times for each.

At the end of the exercises, walk in place for a few minutes. If the leader wishes, other standing exercises from Chapter Nine can be added to the program.

*Neck exercises:*

After the standing exercises, the group may wish to sit down and do some of the neck exercises given in Chapter Ten. Remember that these exercises tend to make you feel drowsy, so be sure the group is seated when you do them.

*Ending the program:*

When I bring my programs to a close, I like to end with a circle dance or a march. Very often I have one group member demonstrate an ethnic dance, and then the rest of the group tries to imitate it—although, of course, it is perfectly all right to substitute your own steps, or just clap or move the hips in time to the music.

If your group is being held in a large hall, you have plenty of room to march around in time to marching music. In a smaller room, you can march in place, although that quickly tires the legs. In the following program to march music, I have suggested ways to alternate other movements with marching so the group doesn't get worn out.

1. Stand straight, behind a chair for balance.

2. Lift legs and march in place in time to the music, to the count of ten.

3. Stop marching. Stretch out arms, palms up. Touch shoulders with hands and stretch arms out again, in time to the music, to the count of five.

4. Bend knees and straighten up, in time to the music, to the count of five.

5. Move hips to the right and then to the left, five times for each side, in time to the music.

6. Clap hands in time to the count of ten.

7. March again in place, to the count of ten.

8. Stretch out hands and open and close fingers to the count of ten.

9. Stretch out arms to the side, and touch shoulders, to the count of five.

10. March again to the count of ten.

If the music isn't finished, and you don't feel tired, repeat some of the activities. However, if at any time any group members feel tired, they should sit down and relax. An individual can also use the marching program at home.

Here is another way to end your program, with an exercise to stimulate the body, the mind, and the memory. You can put this sitting exercise in elsewhere in your program, or you can do it at home.

You start the exercise slowly, and concentrate on not leaving out any part of the body. The object is to stimulate the memory.

1. Put on a lively record with a regular beat. Sit in a chair, with feet firmly on the floor.

2. To the tempo of the music, and using both hands, bend the body and touch shin, knee, thigh, navel, shoulders, head. Raise hands, then touch head, shoulders, navel, thighs, knees, shins. Don't leave out any part of the body.

*After the program:*
Now is the time for the group to sit around and talk. You've put in a good forty-five minutes or hour of exercise, and everyone should feel mentally and physically stimulated.

Laughter and companionship are a good way to end up your sessions. The more fun you have, the more eager everyone will be to stay with the group, and the more devoted to exercise you will be. It will also encourage all participants to keep up their at-home exercising, in order to get more out of the group activities.

## SIXTEEN

# *Education and Exercise*

"*L*OOK at that old man go!" Robert's voice was loud and clear as it rang out over the twenty students in my young people's exercise class.

Lenny, in his seventies, was there in the middle of twenty- and thirty-year-olds, outperforming everyone in the class. Twenty-seven-year-old Robert had just had a rude awakening and a fast education on the value of exercise. Looking at Lenny, Robert saw that his own body, unexercised and already deteriorating, was older than Lenny's. It scared him, and it pushed him into signing up then and there for the class. In a few months, he was keeping up with "that old man." He had learned an important lesson that too few young people learn, or are taught by our society.

I believe that educating the public to the value of exercise is second in importance only to actually doing the exercises. I have proof, in my own life, of the miracles that exercise can perform. Throughout this book, I have given you anecdotes about how exercise has helped many senior citizens in many ways. I hope I have convinced you that an exercise program is a must for older people. But the problem is not just with senior citizens. It has to do with everyone. Young people grow older themselves, whether or not they are willing to admit it in their youth and middle age. And in all those years from childhood through youth, middle age, and old age, there is nothing but ignorance about the significant contribution exercise can make to our health and well-being.

What is the reason for this ignorance? Who are the culprits? Who fails to encourage a lifelong program of exercise, which would make a book like this one unnecessary, because exercise would be a habit instilled in childhood and practiced throughout life?

I blame the educational system that encourages participation in sports, but never informs students fully of the connection between their bodies, their health, and physical activity. I blame the government, which spends millions of dollars to get young people to exercise and rewards those who do, but does not have the foresight to embark on a real educational program that puts exercise in its proper perspective in terms of survival and health in later years. I blame, too, our scientists, researchers and the whole medical profession for failing to support and encourage exercise as a universal form of preventive medicine. How much is prevention worth? Must we always get the disease and then worry about it?

Millions of dollars are spent annually on medical research in areas such as arthritis, cancer, diabetes, heart disease, and even the so-called disease of "old age." I'd like to see equal millions spent on promoting physical fitness. I'd like to see exercise promoted not just as a way to be beautiful, but as a way to remain healthy, active, alert and independent throughout our whole lives.

It must start with the young, and with the schools. It must be made a part of every young person's life, so that as each boy and girl grows up and takes on the responsibilities and pressures of adulthood, exercise is considered a necessary aspect of daily living. Then as those men and women become senior citizens, they still retain the habit of exercise, along with the full understanding of how their physical activities are keeping them healthy and productive human beings.

You, who have read this book and have begun an exercise program in your later years, have a role in this educational process. You can demonstrate the value of exercise for senior citizens. You can do even more: You can use your influence with your families, your children and grandchildren to make them understand what exercise is all about. You can show them what it has done for you, and remind them that one day they, too, will be your age, when every bit of mental and physical fitness keeps life happier and healthier.

You are living proof of the value of exercise. Perhaps from your example the greater questions of money for research, for prevention, for the education of the public will start to be heeded and considered and eventually met and answered, to the lifetime benefit of all our citizens.